Sirtfood Diet

The Complete Guide to Activate Your "Skinny Gene".

It Includes Healthy and Delicious Recipes and a Weekly Weight Loss Plan to Burn Fat, Increase Energy and Improve Your Metabolism Without Fasting or Starving.

Carole J. Lawson

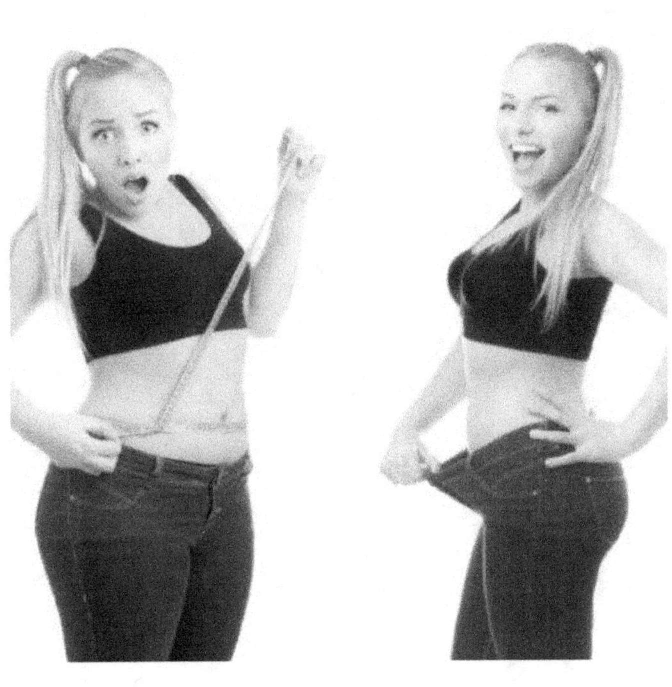

Table of Contents

Introduction

 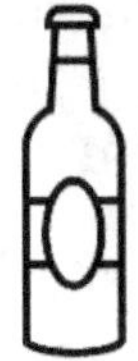 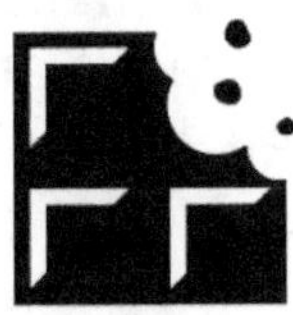

Congratulations on purchasing *Sirtfood,* and thank you for doing so.

The following chapters will discuss the sirtfood diet and what it can do for you. There are so many diet books available today that it is often confusing to know which one is the one that will work for you. But it makes the most sense to choose the eating plan that will allow you to eat the foods you love and still lose weight, simply by adding in specific food choices to your existing diet.

And there is no better diet to choose than the one that has already helped so many people to lose weight. The Sirtfood diet is the obvious choice among both celebrities and non-celebrities. The singer Adele recently used the Sirtfood diet to transform her body into one that is slim and svelte, losing nearly one hundred pounds (forty-five kilos). Champion Olympic sailor Sir Ben Ainslie, model Jodie Kidd, and rugby player James Haskell have all adopted the sirtfood diet to give them the energy and stamina they need for their high profile professions. The diet can be used by models and athletes because it will allow you to lose weight and not muscle mass, where many diets will make you sacrifice one for the other. And with all of these benefits, you will still be able to enjoy flavorful meals made with real foods.

You are taking that first big step toward reaping the benefits of the great new lifestyle plan that everyone is talking about. This is the meal plan that will give you enough energy to make it through your busy day. This is the meal plan that will jump start your weight loss efforts. This is the meal plan you can live with for the remainder of your life and never become bored or unsatisfied.

With all of the books that are available on the market right now on this particular subject, much appreciation for choosing this book. Making certain that it is full of interesting and useful information is a top priority. And if you find this book as helpful as we think you will, please proved a good review on Amazon!

Chapter 1

Sirtfood

What is Sirtfood?

The best new way to lose weight quickly without dieting radically and possibly ruining your health is the Sirtfood diet. This diet works its magic by helping you to activate your skinny gene that is normally only activated by fasting and exercise. The diet emphasizes eating real food like veggies and fruits, fish, and leafy greens that will all help you to lose weight without losing muscle mass or needed energy. You will not be forced to starve in order to lose weight.

Besides the list of the best sirtfoods to eat, the diet plan emphasizes eating healthy, real food. You will use whole foods to prepare your meals and not rely on processed foods and fast foods. The idea is that the sirtfoods will create a reaction in the cells in your body to accelerate your weight loss. The diet depends on caloric restriction along with eating certain foods that will promote good health and weight loss.

What are Sirtuins?

Sirtuins are a select group of proteins that help to regulate the health of your cells, particularly cell homeostasis. In the human body, this means the tendency to keep the internal environment stable and relatively constant. Your body likes its systems and components to be balanced and well-maintained, and sirtuins will help you to do this. A sirtuin is not a dietary protein like those that are found in meat and beans. A sirtuin is the molecule of a protein that carries out many different functions inside of your body. One of their primary jobs in your body is to keep the cells functioning in a balanced, stable way. They do this by using the polyphenols that are found in food that help to activate the sirtuins.

The Purpose of Sirtuins

Sirtuins are the protein enzymes that are in charge of regulating many of the cellular functions in your body, such as circadian rhythms, glucose and fat metabolism, stress resistance, inflammation, and aging. Sirtuins will need the assistance of polyphenols to complete the work they need to do.

The sirtuin proteins have an important role to play in the health of your body. They provide support for many of the cellular processes that are related to your metabolism, like insulin release, the way in which you respond to stress, and how long you and your cells will live. Sirtuin proteins control your circadian rhythms that determine when you wake up and when you sleep. They help to prevent the growth of cancerous cells. Your associative memory, cognitive function, and spatial learning are all improved when your sirtuin proteins are activated. The proteins will prompt your body to use stored fat for energy instead of relying on the increased consumption of food. Sirtuin proteins also govern the rate of metabolism in your cells and how well they respond to hormones, as well as working to decrease inflammation.

So the sirtfoods part of the sirtfood diet is the foods that you will consume that are rich in polyphenols, like red onion, kale, and dark chocolate. These foods work to trigger the sirtuin pathways that have the most effect on mood, aging, and metabolism. You will kick-start your weight loss by consuming foods rich in sirtfoods, and you will maintain optimal health while not losing muscle mass.

This easy-to-follow diet plan will allow you to avoid disease, supercharge your weight loss, and switch on your body's power to burn fat. And merely adding healthy sirtfoods to your diet will help you to sustain weight loss while enjoying glowing health and incredible energy. The sirtfood diet will allow you to include food in your diet, not eliminate them, so it is a diet plan you can remain on for the rest of your life.

The plan emphasizes the particular foods that will awaken the sirtuin activators that are in your body so that you will naturally feel great and lose weight. The idea for this plan came from the minds of two nutritionists who have master's degrees in nutrition. So the diet is based on actual study and research. And while it is a popular diet among celebrities, you don't need to be a celebrity to be successful at this diet.

Chapter 2

The Benefits Of The Sirtfood Diet

The Sirtfood Diet will help you to lose weight, and you might be thinking that weight loss alone is the best possible benefit from the diet. But the weight loss that the diet will make possible will give you so many other health benefits that will get your body back on track to feeling great again. The foods that are the top-recommended foods on the sirtfood list are full of plant compounds that are loaded with nutrients and good for your body. Sirtuin proteins prompt your body to use stored fat for increased energy. This will also help to improve your body's use of the hormone insulin. Besides helping you build muscles and suppress your appetite, the sirtuins will work to improve the function of your brain, help you control your blood sugar, and work to clean up the free radicals that damage the human body. And all this will happen while you are enjoying your foods. Turmeric will add flavor to your foods while it fights inflammation. Dark chocolate helps to fight heart disease, and green tea has long been associated with a reduced risk of stroke and diabetes.

Weight Loss

The best benefit of the sirtfood diet is the ability it gives you to lose weight where you might have failed on so many other diets. Weight loss alone will transform your life because so many of us define ourselves by the way we look. Celebrities certainly do, and that is why so many have turned to this diet. The way you feel about yourself will determine how you carry yourself through the day and interact with the world outside of you. And weight loss will give you so many health benefits.

When people carry excess body weight, their body will create more miles of arteries and veins so they can carry nutrients and oxygen to all parts of the body. These extra miles of arteries cause the heart to pump harder and faster as it attempts to pump the increased need for blood supply, and this can cause you to develop high blood pressure. All of this increased pressure can cause thin spots in the walls of your arteries, and this creates areas for plaque to accumulate. Plaque is nothing more than deposits of calcium, free-floating fat cells, and waste products that have been emitted by your cells. Normally these would be flushed from your body, but when they find a spot to stick to, they will, and this is what makes plaque, which will eventually lead to hardening of the arteries. When this happens, the space in the arteries becomes thin, and the heart will need to work even harder to pump blood. Both of these health problems can eventually lead to the development of cardiovascular disease, which includes strokes and heart attacks.

When you consume food, your pancreas releases the hormone insulin because the brain tells it to do so. Insulin is the compound that will carry the glucose to the cells after your food has been digested. It will carry the glucose to the cells and then gain access for the glucose to enter the cells. Every time you eat, your pancreas makes insulin. When you overeat food, your cells will eventually become full of glucose, and they will stop answering when the insulin comes knocking. When that happens, you have developed what is known as insulin resistance. Then the insulin needs to take the excess glucose somewhere else to store it, and the first place it goes to is your midsection, where the glucose is stored as fat around your internal organs. This is why your midsection is usually the first place to get more significant when you begin to gain weight, and you notice it there because your pants feel tighter. Insulin resistance can lead to metabolic syndrome, which is the collection of excess fat around the stomach area. Having too much glucose, or sugar, floating around in your bloodstream can lead to insulin resistance, which has the potential to lead to the eventual development of Type 2 Diabetes.

Decreased Pain and Inflammation

Another side effect of carrying too much bodyweight is inflammation. Your body will make an area inflamed if it is injured or sick because that is how the body works to support that area while it is healing. Excess weight puts pressure on your joints, particularly the joints in the lower body, and this will cause inflammation. The body perceives that there is an injury because of the pressure of the excess weight, so it will send healing fluids to the sight, which causes swelling and inflammation. Losing weight will lead to a decrease in inflammation.

While it is natural for the body to make inflammation to fight an illness or injury, the wrong kind of inflammation can cause other illnesses to happen. Your body sees no difference between inflammation that happens because of an illness or injury and inflammation that happens because you weigh too much. In either situation the body will send fluids to heal the area and this will cause more inflammation. As you begin to lose weight your body will hurt less and not be as stiff as before, which will automatically decrease your levels of inflammation.

When the inflammation is decreased in your body then you will naturally feel less pain. When excess weight collects around your joints, especially the joints in the lower body, this extra weight will cause stiffness which will lead to pain in the joint. When the brain detects painful feelings it will send fluid to the site to relieve the pain and this excess fluid will cause inflammation. When you lose weight and there is less pressure on your joints, then you will feel less pain and you will experience less inflammation.

Increased Energy and Health

Your cardiovascular system is one of the biggest and most important systems in your body, consisting of the heart, lungs, arteries, and veins. Carrying excess body weight will cause damage to this system, but the effects usually build over time until they become severe health problems, such as hardening of the arteries and high blood pressure. One of the reasons that excess weight causes the heart to work harder is that your body will create extra miles of arteries and veins to be able to carry nutrients to all parts of your body. The increased pressure of the internal walls of the arteries causes thin spots where plaque can collect, and this causes hardening of the arteries. This causes the arteries to narrow and makes the heart work harder to pump blood through the body.

Carrying excess body weight can either cause hormones to run wild or it will depress the hormones that you need to ensure proper metabolism and balance in your body. When the hormones of the body are not produced the way they should be, your body will suffer from several different health issues. Calcium deposits and waste products will build up in your blood and these can cause you to suffer from gout or develop kidney disease. Excess dietary fat can cause the development of kidney stones or stones in the gallbladder. When you use the Sirtfood Diet to lose the excess weight that you are carrying you can alleviate these health issues because you will be getting rid of the underlying problem that caused them.

Whenever you eat your body will produce acids that are secreted into the stomach and intestine for the purpose of digesting your food. When you constantly overeat your body will constantly produce digestive acids. This can lead to ulcers, acid reflux, heartburn, and eventually damage to the esophagus and the lining of the stomach. When you lose weight on the Sirtfood Diet the production of stomach acid will decrease and the damage can eventually reverse itself.

Improved Skin and Hair

Skin is made from a protein known as collagen that your body makes to replenish the skin cells that are aging and dying. Your hair is made of keratin, which carries some of the same amino acids as collagen does. Eventually your body will stop making these compounds. When this happens your hair will begin to thin and may lose its shine, and your skin will begin to sag and wrinkle. These are all inevitable as people get older. But in people who carry excess weight the sirtuin proteins are dormant, and these proteins are needed to keep the body producing collagen and keratin. So when you begin eating sirtfood and the polyphenols activate your sirtuin proteins, your skin will produce more collagen and your hair will produce more keratin. These are the compounds that will keep your hair and skin looking young and healthy longer.

The sirtuin proteins are also thought of as being longevity genes because they will activate and control the compounds in your body that will keep your body operating efficiently for longer periods of time. Sirtfoods are particularly valuable in the fight against aging and all of the issues that come with getting older. There are sirtuin activators in the majority of the plant foods we eat, but certain ones have amounts that are large enough to create a reaction in the body. Sirtuins activate responses that will lead to less cell damage as free radicals are cleansed from your body, and the healthy cells are balanced and able to function correctly. These are the benefits that you will gain from the sirtfood diet without giving up good food and good health.

20

Chapter 3

Phases and Foods of The Sirtfood Diet

The sirtfood diet will give you sustained and effective weight along with glowing health and increased energy. By eating sirtfoods along with your regular diet, you will lose weight almost effortlessly. The diet will help you accomplish this in two phases.

Phases of the Sirtfood Diet

Phase One starts the first day and lasts for one week. During this week, you will limit your daily intake of calories to no more than one thousand. You will eat one meal each day and drink three juices, with the green juice being the most preferred, although other ingredients can be added. You will use ice or water to make the juice smoothies, but you will not use any plant-based milk.

Phase Two begins the second week and lasts for two weeks. Now you will increase your caloric intake if you wish but take in no more than fifteen hundred calories each day. In this phase, you will consume two meals each day and have two juice smoothies.

After finishing Phase Two, you can continue in that phase indefinitely until you have lost the amount of weight that makes you feel the most comfortable in your skin. Or you can begin again with Phase One and keep repeating the cycle until you have lost the weight you desire. Each week you should be able to lose around two to three pounds, which will give you steady weight loss of actual body mass and not accumulated water. All of your excess weight was not gained overnight, and you will not lose it immediately, so stay steady and don't allow yourself to become discouraged. The weight loss will happen.

Top Foods of the Sirtfood Diet

Looking at the foods that are recommended for the sirtfood diet, you will find that these are regular foods that are available in the grocery store or specialty food store. Here is a list of the top sirtfoods and the benefits they will provide you.

Blueberries – The flavonoid that gives blueberries their blue coloring is a powerful antioxidant that will help to prevent the formation of many serious health problems. Blueberries contain vitamin K, zinc, manganese, magnesium, calcium, iron, and phosphorus, all of which are the components found in healthy bones. And vitamin K is needed for calcium absorption. One cup of blueberries will give you twenty-four percent of your daily requirements of vitamin C, which will support the collagen that gives you smooth skin. Blueberries are sodium-free and full of fiber.

Capers – These come from the caper bush, and they are the buds of the immature flowers. After capers are harvested, they are pickled in salty vinegar, and you can use them in sauces, salads, and meat dishes. These will provide a salty, tangy flavor to any dish they are added to. Capers help to stimulate your digestion to help move food through your system faster. They will also help to reduce inflammation in your body and reduce the amount of water retained. Capers are rich in vitamins, fiber, and antioxidants.

Bird's Eye Chilis – These are one of the top ten of the hottest chilies in the world, so you will not need to use much to get flavor for your dishes. Hot chilis have the chemical capsaicin, which is often used in diet pills to help suppress appetite and speed up metabolic processes. It can also help to reduce the spikes in insulin that are associated with insulin resistance. It also increases the production of gastric acid, which will help to move food through your digestive system more quickly by breaking it down faster, thus reducing opportunities for gut damage from slow processes.

Chocolate – Chocolate, especially dark chocolate, is rich with nutrients that can affect your health in positive ways. the seed of the cocoa tree is where chocolate comes from and is a great source of antioxidants. One hundred grams of dark chocolate that is between seventy and eighty-five percent cocoa has almost all of the manganese and copper you need for the day, over half of the magnesium and iron required daily, and eleven grams of fiber. Dark chocolate is loaded with polyphenols. The flavanols can help to improve the lining of your arteries. The antioxidants can help to lower the cholesterol in your arteries that can lead to heart disease, and they can help protect your skin from sun damage and aging.

Cocoa – This food ingredient contains a compound that is an antioxidant that works to reduce your blood pressure and the inflammation in your body. Cocoa is also an anti-inflammatory and can help to reduce your risk of developing heart attacks and strokes. The polyphenols in cocoa activate the sirtuins in your foods. This will work to increase the regular flow of oxygen-rich blood to your brain, which will help to increase its function.

Extra Virgin Olive Oil – All olive oil is good for you, but the extra virgin variety is the best. This type of oil is made by getting the oil from the olives without the use of chemicals or heat, so it is the purest form of all the olive oils available. It is the highest quality of all of the olive oils.

Kale – All leafy greens are good for you, but kale is the king of the greens. As a cruciferous vegetable, it is high in dietary fiber. Eating it regularly will help to lower your blood pressure and relieve the inflammation in your body. Kale helps to cleanse your body of the floating free radicals due to its high level of antioxidants.

Medjool Dates – This is not some exotic form of date but one of the most common varieties available for consumption today. You can buy dates with wrinkled skins, which means they are dried, or smooth skins that tells you they are fresh dates. They will give you dietary fiber, which will help to lower your blood sugar levels and increase activity in your digestive system. They contain antioxidants for your health, particularly carotenoids, which promote eye and heart health. Medjool dates can also help lower your risk of developing chronic illnesses like diabetes, cancer, and Alzheimer's disease because of their high content of flavonoids.

Red Chicory – This is a member of the dandelion family that has been used for centuries in both traditional medicine and kitchen recipes. The root is loaded with prebiotic fiber, which means that it provides all of the health benefits of fiber while also feeding the good bacteria in your gut to help prevent indigestion and bloating. These bacteria also help your gut better absorb the helpful vitamins and minerals in your food. You can grind the roots and use it as a substitute for coffee. You can also boil the whole root and eat it like any other root veggie. The leaves of the plant are a great addition to any salad.

Red Wine – When taken in moderation, a little red wine is good for your health, especially the health of your heart. Red wine has antioxidants that will help protect the lining of your arteries and prevent thin spots where plaque can collect. The resveratrol in red wine promotes the formation of good cholesterol in your blood and also helps to prevent the formation of unhealthy blood clots. The resveratrol in red wine is a natural compound that is found in the skins of grapes, and it will work to lower the levels of sugar in your blood. The antioxidants will work to combat the free radicals in your body that are responsible for every possible disease from the common cold to certain types of cancer. One of the proteins that cause plaque in the brain that can lead to the development of Alzheimer's disease won't grow and develop when red wine is consumed on a regular basis. And red wine helps to block the growth of fat cells.

Soy – Not only is this food the savior of anyone following a vegan diet, but it is also cholesterol free and naturally low in fat content. You will naturally increase your consumption of plant-based protein by including more soy products in your diet like edamame, tofu, and tempeh. Soy is low in carbs and contains vitamins, minerals, and omega-3 fats.

Turmeric – For a nutritional supplement, this spice is probably the best available. Turmeric is the spice that gives the lovely yellow color to foods from the Mediterranean region, particularly curry dishes. For centuries this spice has also been used as both a spice for recipes and an ingredient in traditional medicine, particularly in India. It will help to neutralize the free radicals in your body and naturally reduce inflammation, since it is possibly stronger than many of the anti-inflammatories currently available over the counter.

Walnuts – These carry more antioxidants than any of the other nuts that are edible. They will provide you with healthy fats, fiber, minerals, and vitamins. Walnuts are a good source of vitamin E and polyphenols. Compounds found in walnuts promote a healthy gut, decrease inflammation, and help lower your blood pressure.

Buckwheat – This is a seed and not a wheat product, and it is gluten-free. It is a seed that is loaded with protein and dietary fiber. This is another food item that helps vegans add protein to their diets.

Celery – This crispy veggie has twelve different kinds of antioxidants as well as vitamin C, beta carotene, and flavonoids. It also is a great source of the phytonutrients that will help to reduce inflammation. Celery helps to keep your digestive system functioning properly because it is loaded with dietary fiber.

Coffee – Caffeine is the primary ingredient in coffee, and it is actually full of health benefits. Caffeine will help to suppress your appetite and increase your energy levels because it is a plant-based natural stimulant. Regular consumption will boost your brain functions like memory, reaction times, and mood.

Green Tea – Drinking this beverage regularly will help to promote weight loss. Green tea has minerals, antioxidants, and polyphenols that will help to reduce inflammation and fight cancer. Green tea has enough caffeine to help decrease your appetite, although it contains less caffeine than coffee. And besides helping to hydrate you, it will promote good brain function like vigilance, mood, memory, and reaction time.

Lovage – This is a little-known perennial plant that is easy to grow and has been used for years for medicinal purposes. The stalks are similar in taste and shape to celery, and the leaves resemble cilantro and parsley. Lovage will help to keep your urinary tract healthy since it is a natural diuretic, and it will work to remove excess fluids from your body. Lovage also has antibacterial and anti-inflammatory compounds.

Parsley – This veggie is low in calories, fat, and carbs. One-half cup of parsley will provide you with over one hundred percent of the vitamin A you need daily. You can use parsley as a fresh herb or a dried spice, and it is loaded with antioxidants.

Red Onion – One whole onion has less than fifty calories. Onions carry more than twenty-five different antioxidants, and they are loaded with vitamins and minerals. They will also provide you with most of the B vitamins along with vitamin C and potassium.

Arugula (Rocket) – This veggie is known by both names depending on what part of the world you are in. Arugula is a great addition to smoothies or salads with its distinctive peppery flavor. It has vitamins, minerals, and fiber, and is low in sugar, calories, carbs, and fat. And arugula will help keep you hydrated since it is ninety percent water.

Strawberries – This fruit is low in calories as well as being totally free from sodium, fat, and cholesterol. One serving of this fruit will provide you with more vitamin C than an entire orange, and they are full of fiber, vitamins, and antioxidants. And strawberries are ninety percent water, so they will help with dehydration.

The Benefits of the Sirtfoods

These are the foods that will feature prominently in sirtfood recipes so that you will continue to promote weight loss through the foods you eat. You will use these foods to add to all of the other foods that you make your meals out of to continue your weight loss and good health. While all plant foods contain polyphenols that will activate the sirtuin proteins, these foods have the highest concentration of the polyphenols you need to truly activate your sirtuin proteins and unlock the skinny gene that will aid in your weight loss goals.

When you eat the foods that are high in polyphenols you will easily activate the sirtuin proteins in your cells and see amazing weight loss. Once the sirtuin proteins are activated you will not only enjoy sustained weight loss, but your skin will begin to glow, you will enjoy soaring levels of energy, and your inflammation will decrease.

Since the Sirtfood Diet is not restrictive you will be able to enjoy the foods you like while still eating the sirtfoods that will increase your overall health and help restrict the aging process. It will allow you to develop a lifestyle of healthy eating habits that will carry you throughout the remainder of your life.

Chapter 4

The Green Juice Smoothie

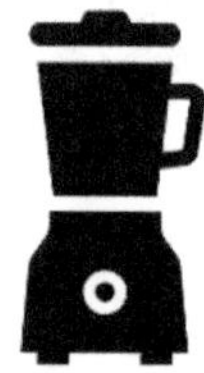

A Dietary Staple

This drink is the one staple of the Sirtfood Diet. This drink by itself is an amazing addition to any diet because it is full of nutrients that your body needs. As this will keep for up to three days in your refrigerator you can make up a large batch of this. Even if you don't want to make larger batches you can definitely make it the night before if time is a factor in your mornings.

Ingredients of the Green Juice Smoothie

The ingredients that the Green Juice Smoothie is made with are loaded with polyphenols that will work to activate your sirtuin proteins in your cells. These chemicals are fund in plant foods and some plants have higher levels of polyphenols than other plants do. The ingredients in the Green Juice Smoothie are all high in different types of polyphenols, so they all work well together to activate your sirtuin proteins. The ingredients are kale, arugula, parsley, celery, green apple, ginger root, lemon juice, and green matcha powder. Everything is blended or juiced together except for the matcha powder and the lemon juice, which you will stir in just before drinking.

Varieties of the Juice Smoothie

While the Green Juice Smoothie is the premier performer on the Sirtfood Diet, many other plant foods can be blended or juiced together to give you a nutrient-rich glass of polyphenols. Chapter Six of this book contains many delicious recipes, and you should feel free to create your own combinations as long as they contain a healthy amount of sirtfoods.

Chapter 5

Sirtfood Diet Meal Plan

This is a sample meal plan for the sirtfood diet that is about to revolutionize your life. There are sample menus for Phase One, which is the first week, and Phase Two, which is weeks two and three. During Phase One, you will consume one thousand calories per day, and during Phase Two, you will consume fifteen hundred calories per day. Feel free to change suggested menu items and make this your own plan. All of the recipes in this meal plan are available in this book.

Calories

Day One
988 calories

Green Smoothie	342
Acai Banana Smoothie	275
Kale and Berry Smoothie	175
Herbed Tomato and Cheese Salad	196

Day Two
948 calories

Green Smoothie	342
Coconut Blueberry Limeade Smoothie	303
Kale Fennel Smoothie	187
Peppers Stuffed with Chicken Salad	116

Day Three
1077 calories

Green Smoothie	342
Blueberry Lime Walnut Smoothie	320
Kale and Berry Smoothie	175
Sloppy Joes	240

Day Four
1026 calories

Walnut Acai Smoothie	250
Mango Blueberry Smoothie	302
Kale and Mushroom Omelet	337
Spicy Kale Scramble	137

Day Five
1010 calories

Banana Walnut Smoothie	295
Avocado Tomato Carrot Smoothie	235
Chicken Cutlet with Chicory Root	300
Baked Fish with Vegetables	180

Day Six
917 calories

Choco Zucchini Smoothie	300
Honeydew Cucumber Smoothie	275
Herbed Omelet with Feta	263
Grilled Chicory Rolls	79

Day Seven
1026 calories

Ginger Carrot and Turmeric Smoothie	310
Green Chili Smoothie	268
Zucchini Noodles with Avocado Sauce	313
Onion and Pepper Pasta	135

Calories

Day One
1386 calories

Green Chili Smoothie	268
Breakfast Salad	336
Hamburger Kale Gratin	350
Beef and Blue Cheese Penne with Pesto	432

Day Two
1355 calories

Pineapple Strawberry Smoothie	286
Roast Tomato Egg White Sandwich	458
Baked Cod with Maple Mustard Sauce	211
Cauliflower Pie	400

Day Three
1164 calories

Berry Beet Mint Smoothie	336
Mediterranean Pasta	267
Portobello Mushroom and Chicory Tacos	405
Indian Roasted Vegetables	156

Day Four
1266 calories

Banana Coffee Cocoa Smoothie	340
Chicken Buckwheat Bowl	432
Salmon with Buckwheat and Vegetables	222
Greek Style Spaghetti Squash	272

Day Five
1235 calories

Walnut Kale Banana Smoothie	319
Kale Avocado and Black Bean Bowl	424
Hasselback Caprese Chicken	355
Grape Tomato and Soba Noodles	137

Day Six
1157 calories

Avocado Kale Pineapple Smoothie	340
Halibut Chowder	262
Philly Cheese Steak	350
Creamy Curry Noodles with Kale	205

Day Seven
1365 calories

Green Smoothie	342
Lamb Stew	389
Korean Steak	350
Tofu in Tomatoes	284

Day Eight
1296 calories

Acai Banana Smoothie	275
Butternut Squash Breakfast Hash	342
Thai Soup	339
Grilled Pork Tenderloin	340

Day Nine
1352 calories

Walnut Acai Smoothie	250
Ham Cheese and Caper Soufflé	460
Egg Roll in a Bowl	178
Shrimp with Lemon and Garlic Pasta	464

Day Ten
1291 calories

Mango Blueberry Smoothie	302
Zucchini Lasagna Rolls	324
Herbed Grilled Cod	275
Feta Chicken Pasta	390

Day Eleven
1174 calories

Kale and Berry Smoothie	175
Salmon with Quinoa and Veggies	298
Buckwheat and Mushroom Risotto	297
Celery and Smoked Sausage Soup	404

Day Twelve
1204 calories

Coconut Blueberry Limeade Smoothie	303
Kale Macaroni Cheese	344
Tuscany Style Vegetables Soup	225
Pesto Pasta	332

Day Thirteen
1143 calories

Kale Fennel Smoothie	187
Sweet Potato and Black Bean Buckwheat Bowl	334
Minestrone	220
Chicken and Avocado Salad	402

Day Fourteen
1258 calories

Banana Walnut Smoothie	295
Avocado Mushroom and Chicory Root Salad	370

So start with these suggestions and then feel free to make the meal plan your own. After you complete the full three weeks, you can continue on with Phase Two or go back to Phase One if you feel you need a jumpstart to accelerated weight loss. And any time you feel your journey needs a boost, just start over with Phase One.

And if you are enjoying the book so far a good review on Amazon will be greatly appreciated!

Chapter 6

Juice Smoothie Recipes

The juice or smoothie is a staple of the sirtfood diet, particularly the Green Smoothie that is the main recipe of the sirtfood diet recipes. Any smoothie can be loaded with nutrients that will give you amazing health benefits as well as keeping you full and well-hydrated. Smoothies can be made in a blender, but a juicer is the better option. You can also make smoothies in large enough amounts to keep them in the refrigerator so that you can make one batch in the morning and have it available all day.

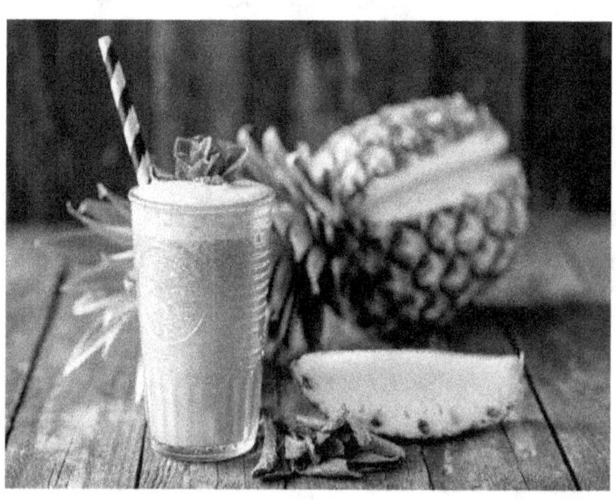

Green Smoothie Recipe

342 Calories in eight ounces

Ingredients:

Matcha green tea, one-half teaspoon
Arugula, one-fourth cup
Kale, three-fourths cup
Lemon juice, one tablespoon
Ginger, ground, one teaspoon
Green apple, one-half of one
Celery, two stalks
Parsley, chopped, one-fourth cup

Juice or blend all of the ingredients together except for the lemon juice and the matcha green tea. When you have all of the ingredients blended together well, you can then stir in the matcha green tea and the lemon juice by hand. Drink eight ounces for one serving.

Acai Banana Smoothie

275 Calories in eight ounces

Ingredients:

Matcha green tea, one teaspoon
Lime juice, one tablespoon
Coconut water, one cup
Kale, chopped, one-half cup
Blueberries, frozen, one-half cup
Mango, frozen, one-half cup
Banana, frozen, one

Walnut Acai Smoothie

250 Calories in eight ounces

Ingredients:

Walnut butter, two tablespoons
Whey protein powder, vanilla, two scoops
Strawberries, frozen and sliced, one cup
Coconut water, one cup
Acai berries, one-half cup

Mango Blueberry Smoothie

302 Calories in eight ounces

Ingredients:

Turmeric, ground, one-half teaspoon
Coconut water, one cup
Blueberries, frozen, one-half cup
Banana, frozen, one
Mango, frozen, one peeled and chopped

Kale and Berry Smoothie

175 Calories in eight ounces

Ingredients:

Strawberries, six
Blueberries, frozen, one-half cup
Kale, fresh, one-fourth cup
Ginger, ground, one-half teaspoon
Turmeric, one-half teaspoon
Apple juice, unsweetened, one half cup
Lemon juice, one tablespoon

Coconut Blueberry Limeade Smoothie

303 Calories in eight ounces

Ingredients:

Cold water, one-half cup
Coconut milk, one-half cup
Blueberries, three-fourths cup
Cherries, pitted, one cup
Banana, frozen, one-half of one
Lime juice, one tablespoon

Kale Fennel Smoothie

187 Calories in eight ounces

Ingredients:

Lime juice, two tablespoons
Apple juice, unsweetened, one-half cup
Kale, chopped, one-half cup
Fennel, chopped, one-half cup
Coconut water, one-half cup
Ginger, ground, one teaspoon
Turmeric, ground, one teaspoon
Celery, chopped, one-half cup

Blueberry Lime Walnut Smoothie

320 Calories in eight ounces

50

Ingredients:

Lime juice, two tablespoons
Coconut water, two cups
Blueberries, fresh or frozen, one cup
Walnuts, chopped, one cup
Medjool dates, three pitted and chopped

Banana Walnut Smoothie

295 Calories in eight ounces

Ingredients:

Vanilla extract, one teaspoon
Walnuts butter, two tablespoons
Coconut water, one cup
Banana, frozen, two

Avocado Tomato Carrot Smoothie

235 Calories in eight ounces

52

Ingredients:

Cold water, one cup
Cayenne pepper, one-eighth teaspoon
Tomato, one medium chopped
Kale, chopped, one cup
Garlic, minced, one teaspoon
Lime juice, two tablespoons
Cucumber, peeled and seeded, one-half of one
Carrot, one medium chopped

Choco Zucchini Smoothie

300 Calories in eight cups

Ingredients:

Coconut water, chilled, one cup
Cocoa powder, two tablespoons
Turmeric, ground, one teaspoon
Blueberries, frozen, one-half cup
Banana, frozen, one large
Zucchini, frozen, grated, one cup
Red chicory, chopped, one-half cup

Honeydew Cucumber Smoothie

275 Calories in eight ounces

Ingredients:

Cucumber, chilled or frozen, three-fourths cup
Lime juice, two tablespoons
Coconut water, two cups
Honeydew, chilled and chunked, two cups
Turmeric, ground, one teaspoon
Ginger, ground, one teaspoon

Ginger Carrot and Turmeric Smoothie

310 Calories in eight ounces

Ingredients:

Turmeric, ground, one teaspoon
Ginger, ground, one teaspoon
Hemp Seeds, raw, one tablespoon
Coconut water, one cup
Navel orange, one peeled and sectioned
Carrot, one peeled and chunked

Avocado Kale Pineapple Smoothie

340 Calories in eight ounces

Ingredients:

Matcha green tea powder, one tablespoon
Lemon juice, two tablespoons
Coconut water, one cup
Coconut, unsweetened and shredded, one-half cup
Pineapple chunks, unsweetened, frozen, one-half cup
Kale, chopped, one-half cup
Avocado, peeled and pitted, one

Green Chili Smoothie

268 Calories in eight ounces

Ingredients:

Lime juice, one tablespoon
Mint, chopped, two tablespoons
Coconut water, one cup
Kale, chopped, one-half cup
Parsley, chopped, one-fourth cup
Jalapeno, chopped, one tablespoon
Cucumber, seeded and chopped, one cup

Pineapple Strawberry Smoothie

286 Calories in eight ounces

58

Ingredients:

Turmeric, ground, one teaspoon
Ginger, ground, one teaspoon
Coconut water, two cups
Strawberries, sliced, one cup
Pineapple chunks, frozen, two cups

286 Calories in eight ounces

Berry Beet Mint Smoothie

336 Calories in eight ounces

Ingredients:

Chia seeds, ground, one tablespoon
Lime juice, two tablespoons
Mint leaves, one-fourth cup
Beet, grated, one-fourth cup
Blueberries, frozen, one cup
Coconut water, one cup

Banana Coffee Cocoa Smoothie

340 Calories in eight ounces

60

Ingredients:

Cinnamon, one teaspoon
Cocoa powder, unsweetened, one tablespoon
Walnuts, chopped, one-fourth cup
Coffee, cold, one-half cup
Medjool dates, chopped, two
Banana, frozen, one

Walnut Kale Banana Smoothie

319 Calories in eight ounces

Ingredients:

Coconut water, one cup
Kale, chopped, two cups
Banana, frozen, one
Walnuts, chopped, one-fourth cup
Medjool dates, chopped, two
Orange, one peeled and sectioned

Parsley Kale Berry Smoothie

302 Calories in eight ounces

Ingredients:

Flaxseed, ground, one teaspoon
Banana, frozen, one
Strawberries, frozen and sliced, one cup
Kale, chopped, one-half cup
Turmeric, ground, one teaspoon
Cinnamon, ground, one teaspoon
Parsley, chopped, one-half cup

Avocado Parsley Lime Smoothie

337 Calories in eight ounces

Ingredients:

Parsley, chopped, one-fourth cup
Lime juice, two tablespoons
Coconut water, one cup
Avocado, one peeled and pitted
Turmeric, ground, one teaspoon

Berry Pomegranate Smoothie

165 Calories in eight ounces

Ingredients:

Lime juice, one tablespoon
Pomegranate juice, one-fourth cup
Ginger, ground, one teaspoon
Beets, cooked and chopped, one-fourth cup
Rhubarb, chopped, one-half cup
Strawberries, frozen, one-fourth cup
Celery, chopped, one-fourth cup

Apple Cinnamon Smoothie

149 Calories in eight ounces

Ingredients:

Cinnamon, one teaspoon
Spinach, fresh, chopped, one cup
Apple, red or green, sliced and cored, one
Pear, cored and sliced, one
Apple juice, unsweetened, one cup

Blueberry Pumpkin Spice Smoothie

280 Calories in eight ounces

Ingredients:

Ginger, one-half teaspoon
Cloves, ground, one-half teaspoon
Banana, frozen, one
Coconut water, one cup
Cinnamon, ground, one teaspoon
Blueberry, frozen, one-half cup
Nutmeg, ground, one teaspoon
Vanilla extract, one teaspoon
Vanilla protein powder, one scoop
Medjool dates, two pitted
Pumpkin, pureed, one-half cup

Orange Blueberry Smoothie

355 Calories in eight ounces

Ingredients:

Blueberries, frozen, one-half cup
Orange, one small peeled and sectioned
Cold water, one cup
Vanilla extract, one teaspoon
Cinnamon, ground, one teaspoon

Chapter 7

Recipes For Breakfast

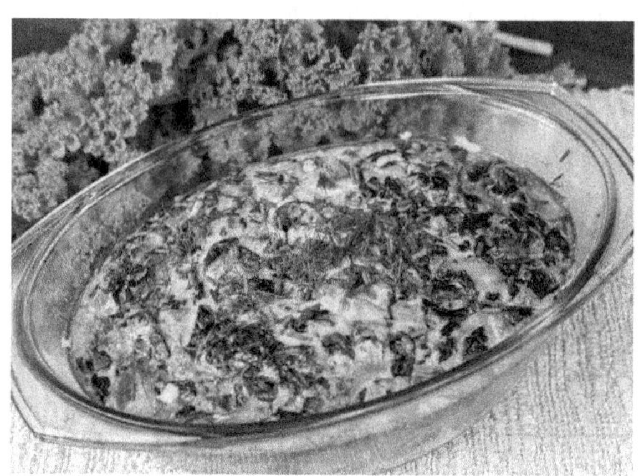

Kale and Mushroom Omelet

Prep three min/cook fifteen min/serves one to two/calories 337
Gluten-free and Vegan (use nutritional yeast instead of feta cheese)

Ingredients:

- Feta cheese, one ounce

- Kale, fresh, chopped, one and one half cup
- Green onion, three diced
- Eggs, three
- Mushrooms, button, five sliced
- Extra virgin olive oil, two tablespoons divided
- Red onion, diced, one quarter cup

Instructions:

Over medium heat warm one tablespoon of the olive oil and fry the kale, onions, and mushrooms for five minutes. Remove these from the skillet and set them off to the side. Add the remainder of the olive oil to the hot skillet. Beat the eggs well in a smaller bowl, and then pour them into the skillet, allowing them to spread across the bottom completely. Let the eggs fry undisturbed for five minutes, or until the outer one inch has cooked and looks dry. Pour the fried ingredients into the part of the omelet that is still wet and then fold one half over the other half. Let the omelet cook for three more minutes and then flip it over and cook it for three more minutes on the other side.

**Breakfast Salad**

Prep thirty min/serves four/calories 336
Gluten-free

Ingredients:

- Eggs, four hard-boiled and sliced
- Lemon, one
- Arugula, ten cups
- Buckwheat, one cup cooked and cooled
- Extra virgin olive oil, two tablespoons
- Parsley, chopped, one-half cup
- Walnuts, chopped, one cup
- Avocado, one large sliced thin
- Celery, chopped, one-half cup
- Tomato, one large cut in wedges

Instructions:

Blend together in a large-sized bowl the arugula with the cooked buckwheat, tomatoes, and celery, tossing them together gently until they are well mixed. Divide the salad mix on four serving plates and lay the slices of avocado and boiled egg on top. Use the herbs and walnuts to garnish the top of each salad.

Spicy Kale Scramble

Prep five min/cook ten min/serves one/calories 137
Gluten-free

Ingredients:

- Extra virgin olive oil, two tablespoons
- Sprouts, any type, one-half cup
- Black pepper, one-fourth teaspoon
- Turmeric, ground, one tablespoon
- Garlic, minced, one tablespoon
- Kale, shredded, one-half cup
- Eggs, two
- Bird's Eye chili, chopped, one tablespoon

Instructions:

Beat the eggs with the garlic, black pepper, and turmeric in a medium-sized bowl. Fry the kale in the olive oil over medium heat for five minutes, and then pour the mixture of egg into the kale. Continue cooking while you stir constantly to cook the eggs to the desired degree of scrambled doneness. Top the eggs with the chopped chili and raw sprouts and serve.

Egg Muffins With Quinoa and Feta Cheese

Prep fifteen min/cook thirty min/serves six/calories 226
Gluten-free

Ingredients:

- Eggs, eight
- Tomatoes, chopped, one cup
- Sea salt, one-fourth teaspoon
- Feta cheese, one cup
- Quinoa, one cup cooked
- Extra virgin olive oil, two teaspoons
- Oregano, fresh chop, one tablespoon
- Parsley, chopped, one-fourth cup
- Black olives, chopped, one-fourth cup
- Red onion, chopped, one-fourth cup
- Kale, chopped, two cups
- Olive oil spray oil

Instructions:

Heat your oven to 350. Use the spray to grease a muffin cup pan with twelve cups. Fry the olives, onion, kale, oregano, and tomatoes for five minutes in the olive oil using medium heat. Beat the eggs in a larger sized bowl. Pour the mixture of cooked veggies into the eggs with the cheese and salt. Place the mix into the muffin cups, dividing the mixture evenly between all twelve cups. Bake the egg muffins for thirty minutes. These will remain edibly fresh in the fridge for two days. To eat the next day, just wrap the egg muffin in a paper towel and warm it in the microwave for thirty seconds.

Buckwheat Breakfast Bowl

Prep thirty minutes/serves six/calories 340
Gluten-free

Ingredients:

- Buckwheat, two cups cooked
- Sea salt, one-half teaspoon
- Eggs, twelve
- Greek yogurt, plain and unsweetened, one quarter cup
- Black pepper, one teaspoon
- Feta cheese, one cup
- Cherry tomatoes, one pint cut in halves
- Extra virgin olive oil, one teaspoon
- Garlic, minced, one teaspoon
- Kale, chopped, one cup

Instructions:

Mix together in a large-sized bowl the garlic, onion powder, eggs, salt, pepper, and yogurt. Fry the kale and tomatoes for five minutes in the olive oil over medium heat. Pour in the egg mix to the skillet and stir until the eggs have set to your preferred doneness. Mix in the buckwheat and feta until they are hot. This will store in the fridge for two to three days.

Mediterranean Frittata

Prep five minutes/cook twenty minutes/serves six/calories 107
Gluten-free

Ingredients:

- Eggs, six
- Feta cheese, crumbled, one quarter cup
- Black pepper, one-fourth teaspoon
- Oregano, one teaspoon
- Sea salt, one teaspoon
- Black olives, chopped, one-fourth cup
- Green olives, chopped, one-fourth cup
- Tomatoes, diced, one quarter cup
- Milk, almond or coconut, one-fourth cup
- Olive oil spray oil

Instructions:

Heat the oven to 400. Use the spray oil to grease an eight by eight-inch baking dish. In a medium-sized mixing bowl, beat the milk into the eggs and then add the salt, pepper, oregano, tomatoes, black olives, and green olives. Pour all of this mixture into the baking dish and sprinkle the feta cheese on top, and bake the frittata for twenty minutes.

Maple Nut Buckwheat

Prep five min/cook twenty min/serves four/calories 374
Gluten-free and vegan

Ingredients:

- Maple flavoring, one teaspoon
- Cinnamon, one teaspoon
- Almonds, chopped, three tablespoons
- Pecans, one-half cup chopped
- Walnuts, one-half cup chopped
- Chia seeds, four tablespoons
- Milk, almond or coconut, one-half cup
- Coconut flakes, unsweetened, one-fourth cup

Instructions:

Pulse the walnuts, almonds, and pecans in a food processor to crumble. Or you can just put the nuts in a sturdy plastic bag, wrap the bag with a towel, lay it on a sturdy surface, and beat the towel with a hammer until the nuts are crumbled. Mix the crushed nuts with the rest of the ingredients in the list in a larger size saucepot. Simmer this over low heat for thirty minutes. Stir the buckwheat often, so the mix does not stick to the bottom. Serve garnished with fresh fruit or a sprinkle of cinnamon if desired.

**Tomato Omelet**

Prep two min/cook eight min/serves one/calories 342
Gluten-free

Ingredients:

- Eggs, two
- Parsley, fresh, one-half cup
- Cherry tomatoes, one-half cup
- Black pepper, one teaspoon
- Sea salt, one-half teaspoon
- Nutritional yeast, one-half cup
- Turmeric, ground, one teaspoon
- Ginger, ground, one teaspoon
- Extra virgin olive oil, two tablespoons

Instructions:

Cut the tomatoes into quarters and fry them in hot olive oil for four minutes. Set the tomatoes off to one side to drain. In a smaller bowl, put pepper and salt into the eggs and beat together well. Pour the beaten mixture of egg into the pan and use a spatula to gently work around the edges under the omelet, letting the eggs fry unmoved for three minutes. When just the center third of the egg mix is still runny, add in the parsley, tomatoes, and nutritional yeast. Fold over half of the omelet onto the other half. Cook three more minutes and serve.

Tofu Scramble With Curry

Prep ten minutes/cook twenty minutes/serves four/calories 118
Gluten-free and vegan

Ingredients:

- SCRAMBLE
- Kale, roughly chopped, three cups
- Red onion, diced, one-half medium
- Extra virgin olive oil, one tablespoon
- Tofu, firm, eight-ounce block
- Mushrooms, sliced, six ounces
- Red bell pepper, diced and cleaned, one large

- SAUCE
- Garam masala, one-fourth teaspoon
- Turmeric, ground, one-fourth teaspoon
- Paprika, ground, one-fourth teaspoon
- Coriander, ground, one-fourth teaspoon
- Cumin, ground, one-fourth teaspoon
- Garlic powder, one-fourth teaspoon
- Curry powder, one-fourth teaspoon

Instructions:

Press the block of tofu between paper towels for thirty minutes to remove the excess liquid before beginning the recipe to remove all of the excess liquid in the block. For five minutes, fry the onion by itself in the hot oil, and then put in the red peppers and the sliced mushrooms and cook for an additional ten minutes. Push the cooked vegetables to one half of the skillet and put the tofu in the other half, breaking it into little chunks. Cook the tofu for five minutes. While the tofu is cooking, put all of the seasoning ingredients into a bowl and whip them together. Sprinkle this mixture over the ingredients in the skillet and mix it all together. Add in the greens and cook this for five more minutes, and then serve.

Egg Toast With Poached Salmon

Prep ten min/cook four min/serves two/calories 389

Ingredients:

- Bread, two slices rye or whole-grain toasted
- Lemon juice, one-fourth teaspoon
- Avocado, mashed, two tablespoons
- Black pepper, one-fourth teaspoon
- Eggs, two poached
- Salmon, smoked, four ounces
- Red onions, sliced thinly, one-fourth cup
- Parsley, chopped, one-fourth cup

Instructions:

Add the lemon juice to the mashed avocado and stir in the pepper. Spread the avocado mixture over the toasted slices of bread. Lay the smoked salmon over the toast and top each slice with a poached egg. Top everything with the sliced red onions and chopped parsley.

Veggie Breakfast Burrito

Prep fifteen min/ cook five min/serves six/calories 252
Vegan

Ingredients:

- Extra virgin olive oil, two tablespoons
- Tortillas, ten-inch size, low carb, six
- Black olives, sliced, three tablespoons
- Tomatoes, chopped, three tablespoons
- Nutritional yeast, one half of one cup
- Red onion, thinly sliced, one-fourth teaspoon
- Kale, two cups, washed and dried
- Refried beans, canned, three-fourths of one cup
- Salsa for garnish

Instructions:

Fry the kale, black olives, and tomatoes in a large skillet in the olive oil for five minutes while you are stirring constantly. Put two tablespoons of the refried beans on each of the tortillas and spread it over the tortillas, going to just one inch from the edge. Divide the veggie mixture evenly over the tortillas and sprinkle on the nutritional yeast. Roll each one up by folding the sides in and then rolling the tortilla. Place the burritos back in the skillet with the leftover olive oil and fry the rolled burritos for three minutes on each side. Serve them with the salsa if desired.

Cinnamon Buckwheat Bowl

Prep five min/cook fifteen min/serves two/calories 265
Gluten-free and vegan

Ingredients:

- Strawberries, sliced, one cup
- Vanilla extract, one teaspoon
- Cinnamon, one teaspoon
- Almond milk, one cup
- Water, one cup
- Buckwheat groats, one cup rinsed

Instructions:

Add the vanilla extract, cinnamon, almond milk, water, and buckwheat groats to a medium-sized saucepan and set it over medium heat. Let the mix start to boil, and then lower the temperature and let the buckwheat simmer for ten minutes while partially covered. Remove the saucepan from the heat and completely cover it, and then let the buckwheat steam for five more minutes. Fluff the buckwheat with a fork and then divide it into two serving bowls and top each bowl with half of the sliced strawberries.

Sweet Potato Hash Egg Muffin

Prep ten min/cook fifteen min/serves eight/calories 103
Gluten-free

Ingredients:

- Sea salt, one-half teaspoon
- Black pepper, one teaspoon
- Eggs, eight
- Garlic powder, one-half tablespoon
- Cheddar cheese, shredded, one-half cup
- Sweet potato or yam, one small, grated
- Olive oil spray oil
- Parsley, finely chopped, one-fourth cup
- Turmeric, one teaspoon

Instructions:

Heat the oven to 375. Use the olive oil spray to grease eight of the cups of a twelve cup muffin pan. The sweet potato or yam can be easily grated on a cheese grater or in a food processor. After it is grated, then place it in a larger size bowl and blend in the parsley, black pepper, garlic powder, turmeric, and cheddar cheese. Place one tablespoon of this mix in each of eight cups in the muffin pan. Then break one egg into each cup. Bake these for twelve to sixteen minutes or until the egg is cooked the way you prefer.

Buckwheat Berry Pancakes

Prep fifteen min/cook ten min/serves three to four/calories 150 (four cakes)
Gluten-free and vegan

Ingredients:

- Extra virgin olive oil, two tablespoons
- Milk, coconut or almond, one and one-half cups
- Turmeric, ground, three teaspoons
- Cardamom, ground, one-half teaspoon
- Vanilla extract, one teaspoon
- Baking powder, one teaspoon
- Banana, one
- Buckwheat flour, two cups
- Blueberries, fresh or thawed frozen, unsweetened, one cup

Instructions:

Mash the banana until smooth and then blend in the milk and vanilla. In a separate large bowl, mix the baking powder, buckwheat flour, cardamom, and turmeric just until blended. Add in the wet ingredients and stir gently just until the two are well mixed. Use two tablespoons of batter for each pancake and cook them in the hot oil. Cook each pancake for three to four minutes or until the top is mostly covered with bubbles and then flip to cook on the other side. Serve the pancakes with the blueberries on top.

Kale Mozzarella Frittata

Prep fifteen min/cook twenty min/serves four to six/calories 315
Gluten-free

Ingredients:

- Mozzarella cheese, shredded, one cup
- Red onion, diced, one-half cup
- Kale, one cup diced
- Almond milk, one half cup
- Eggs, eight
- Extra virgin olive oil, two tablespoons
- Olive oil spray oil

Instructions:

Heat the oven to 450. Fry the kale and the red onions in the olive oil for five minutes over medium heat. While they are frying, beat the eggs and milk in a medium-sized bowl. Use the spray oil to grease a nine-inch baking pan and pour the onion and kale mixture into it. Pour the eggs over the spinach mix and cover the eggs with the shredded cheese. Bake the frittata for twenty minutes.

Spicy Skillet Eggs

Prep five min/cook ten min/serves two/calories 620
Gluten-free

Ingredients:

- Parmesan cheese, grated, one-fourth cup
- Extra virgin olive oil, one tablespoon
- Mozzarella cheese, six ounces shredded
- Diced tomatoes, one twenty-eight ounce can
- Turmeric, ground, one teaspoon
- Garlic, minced, two tablespoons
- Eggs, four
- Black pepper, one-half teaspoon
- Bird's eye chili, diced finely, one-fourth teaspoon

Instructions:

Fry the garlic and bird's eye chili in the olive oil for two minutes over medium heat. Pour in the can of tomatoes with the juice and then stir in the turmeric and pepper. Simmer until the mix begins to bubble, and then cook it for five more minutes. Make four holes with the back of a spoon and crack one egg into each of the wells. Sprinkle both kinds of cheese over the mix and cook for ten minutes.

Peppers and Onions With Scramble Tofu

Prep five min/cook five min/serves two/calories 369
Gluten-free and vegan

Ingredients:

- Tofu, extra firm, eight ounces
- Extra virgin olive oil, one tablespoon
- Parsley, fresh, one-third cup
- Black pepper, one teaspoon
- Red onion, diced, one-half cup
- Cheddar cheese, shredded, one-half cup or nutritional yeast, one half cup
- Red bell pepper, one diced

Instructions:

Fry the chopped peppers and red onions in the olive oil for five minutes over medium heat. While they are frying, squeeze the excess liquid out of the tofu and break it up into small chunks. Add the chunks of tofu to the onions and peppers in the skillet and scramble until they are warmed through, for about six minutes, while you are stirring often. Stir the cheese or nutritional yeast with the parsley into the tofu mixture, mix well and serve.

Quiche Cups

Prep ten min/cook thirty min/makes twelve cups/calories 67
Gluten-free and vegan

Ingredients:

- Cornstarch, one tablespoon
- Tomato paste, one tablespoon
- Water, three tablespoons
- Nutritional yeast, one-half cup
- Olive oil spray oil
- Dijon mustard, two tablespoons
- Turmeric, one teaspoon
- Black pepper, one teaspoon
- Tofu, extra firm, one block (fourteen ounces)
- Garlic powder, two teaspoons
- Kale, frozen and thawed, four cups
- Lemon juice, one tablespoon

Instructions:

Heat the oven to 350. Use the spray oil to grease all of the cups of a twelve cup muffin pan and set it to the side. Blend together all of the ingredients listed into a blender except for the kale and blend them on high until the mixture is smooth and creamy. Put the kale into a large bowl and then pour the mix from the blender into the bowl. Stir the liquid mix together with the kale and then divide this mix into the twelve muffin cups, making them as even as possible.

Bake the muffins for thirty to thirty-five minutes or until just the edges are turning slightly brown.

Strawberry French Toast

Prep ten min/cook forty-five min/serves eight/calories 200

Ingredients:

- Maple syrup or plain Greek yogurt for topping
- Sea salt, one-fourth teaspoon
- Cinnamon, ground, one teaspoon
- Vanilla extract, one tablespoon
- Eggs, six large
- Almond milk, one cup
- Cornstarch, one tablespoon
- Honey, one-third cup
- Strawberries, one pint rinsed and sliced
- Sourdough bread, eight slices
- Olive oil pan spray

Instructions:

Pour the strawberries in a mixing bowl and blend them with the honey and cornstarch. Cut or tear the slices of sourdough bread into cubes one inch in size and set them to the side. In a different medium-sized mixing bowl, blend together the cinnamon, vanilla extract, milk, and eggs until they are mixed well together. Use the spray oil to grease a thirteen by nine-inch baking dish and put one-third of the strawberries into the serving dish. Dump the mixture of egg over the strawberries. Dot the remainder of the strawberries over the egg mix and cover the dish with plastic wrap. Set the dish in the refrigerator for a minimum of four hours, although overnight is better. When the time comes to bake the casserole, heat the oven to 375 and remove the plastic wrap from the casserole whiles the oven heats. Remove the plastic wrap and bake the casserole for forty-five minutes. Let it cool for ten minutes after you pull the casserole from the oven before serving with the maple syrup or Greek yogurt.

Chocolate Chip Strawberry Buckwheat Pancakes

Prep five min/cook thirty min/makes four/calories 175
Gluten-free and vegan

Ingredients:

- Dark chocolate chips, one-fourth cup
- Strawberries, chopped, one-half cup
- Applesauce, one-half cup
- Vanilla extract, one tablespoon
- Extra virgin olive oil, two tablespoons
- Almond milk, unsweetened, three-fourths cup
- Sea salt, one-fourth teaspoon
- Cinnamon, ground, one teaspoon
- Baking powder, one teaspoon
- Agave nectar, two tablespoons
- Buckwheat flour, one cup
- Olive oil spray oil

Instructions:

Use the spray oil to grease a large skillet and heat it over medium heat. Use a large size mixing bowl to blend together the buckwheat flour with the salt, cinnamon, and baking powder. In a smaller mixing bowl, mix the agave nectar, vanilla extract, olive oil, and almond milk until they are well blended. Fold the milk mix into the mixture of flour, stirring gently until all of the ingredients are barely blended. Then gently fold the chocolate chips and the strawberries in. Use one-half cup of batter to make a five to six-inch pancake in the skillet, cooking each pancake for five to six minutes on each side.

Herbed Omelet With Feta

Prep ten min/cook ten min/serves two/calories 263
Gluten-free

Ingredients:

- Sea salt, one-half teaspoon
- Lemon juice, one tablespoon
- Black pepper, one teaspoon
- Feta cheese, crumbled, one-fourth cup
- Kale, chopped, one-half cup
- Eggs, four
- Extra virgin olive oil, one tablespoon
- One teaspoon each of dried parsley, chopped mint, tarragon, basil, and rosemary

Instructions:

Beat the herbs together with the eggs and the salt and pepper. Pour in the egg mixture into the heated oil in a large skillet and let it completely cover the bottom, and then cook it undisturbed for three minutes. Gently drag a spatula through the center of the egg to let the runny part leak into the pan and cook. When most of the omelet is set, sprinkle the kale and feta cheese over half of the omelet and then flip the other half over it. Cook the omelet for two minutes more and then drizzle with the lemon juice.

Roasted Tomato Egg White Sandwich

Prep ten min/cook twenty min/serves one/calories 458

Ingredients:

- Egg whites, one-half cup
- Red onion, two slices
- Parsley, chopped, one teaspoon
- Ciabatta roll, one
- Provolone cheese, two slices
- Tomato, two slices
- Extra virgin olive oil, one tablespoon

Instructions:

Slice the ciabatta roll in half through the middle and toast both halves. Warm the oil in a medium-sized skillet over medium heat and fry the tomato slices for three minutes on each side. Place the slices of cheese on the toasted ciabatta roll halves. Remove the tomato slices from the skillet and fry the egg whites until they are done. Divide the egg whites and place them on top of the provolone cheese, and then add on the onion slices and the tomato slices. Sprinkle the top with the chopped parsley and enjoy.

Blueberry Banana Muffins

Prep twenty min/cook twenty-five min/serves twelve/calories 180
Gluten-free and Vegan

Ingredients:

- Banana, one mashed
- Almond milk, three-fourths cup
- Apple cider vinegar, one teaspoon
- Maple syrup, one-fourth cup
- Vanilla extract, one teaspoon
- Extra virgin olive oil, one-fourth cup
- Buckwheat flour, two cups
- Agave nectar, four tablespoons
- Baking powder, two teaspoons
- Cinnamon, ground, two teaspoons
- Sea salt, one-half teaspoon
- Baking soda, one-half teaspoon
- Walnuts, chopped, one-half cup
- Blueberries, fresh, two cups
- Olive oil spray oil

Instructions:

Heat the oven to 350. Use the spray oil to grease all twelve cups of a twelve cup muffin pan. Mash the banana and put it in a medium-sized mixing bowl. Next, you will blend in the almond milk, vinegar, agave nectar, maple syrup, and vanilla. Blend the buckwheat flour in a larger mixing bowl with the baking powder, baking soda, cinnamon, and salt. Blend the mixture with the almond milk into the mixture of the flour, folding over gently just until the drier ingredients are completely moistened. Gently fold in the walnuts and blueberries. Place the batter into the muffin cups, dividing it evenly among the twelve cups. Bake the muffins for twenty-five minutes.

Butternut Squash Breakfast Hash

Prep ten min/cook ten min/serves two/calories 342
Gluten-free

Ingredients:

- Sea salt, one-half teaspoon
- Black pepper, one teaspoon
- Egg, four fried
- Kale, chopped, one-half cup
- Garlic, minced, one tablespoon
- Lemon juice, one tablespoon
- Parsley, chopped, two tablespoons
- Broccoli florets, one cup
- Zucchini, one small sliced thin
- Red onion, diced, one-fourth cup
- Extra virgin olive oil, one tablespoon
- Butternut squash, cubes, two cups
- Olive oil spray oil

Instructions:

Heat the oven to 400. Use the spray oil to coat a baking pan and set the cubes of butternut squash on the oiled baking pan. Roast the squash for thirty minutes. After the squash has roasted, set a larger skillet over medium heat and fry in hot oil the red onion, broccoli, parsley, and zucchini with the salt and pepper for eight minutes, stirring occasionally. Add in the lemon juice, butternut squash, garlic, and kale and cook all of this together for five more minutes. Divide this mixture onto two serving plates and top each plate with two fried eggs.

Chocolate Zucchini Bread

Prep fifteen min/cook forty-five min/serves sixteen/calories 329

Ingredients:

- Baking powder, one tablespoon
- Dark chocolate chips, one cup
- Baking soda, one teaspoon
- Zucchini, unpeeled and shredded, two cups
- Sea salt, one teaspoon
- Vanilla extract, two teaspoons
- Extra virgin olive oil, one-fourth cup
- Maple syrup, two-thirds cup
- Cinnamon, one teaspoon
- Almond milk, one and one-half cups
- Applesauce, unsweetened, one-half cup
- Nutmeg, one-half teaspoon
- Cocoa powder, one-third cup
- Buckwheat flour, two and one-half cups
- Olive oil pan spray

Instructions:

Heat the oven to 350. Use the spray oil to grease two loaf pans and set them to the side. In a medium-sized bowl, blend together the cocoa powder, nutmeg, baking powder, cinnamon, salt, baking soda, and the buckwheat flour. In a large-sized mixing bowl, mix the vanilla, maple syrup, applesauce, olive oil, and almond milk and then pour the flour mixture into this gradually while mixing well. Gently fold in the chocolate chips and the zucchini. Spoon the mixture evenly between the two loaf pans and bake the loaves for forty-five minutes.

Chapter 8

Recipes For Lunch

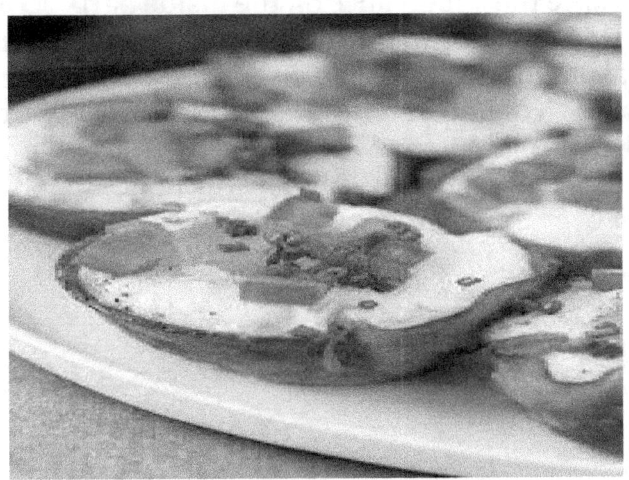

Herbed Tomato and Cheese Salad

Prep ten min/serves four/calories 196
Gluten-free

Ingredients:

- Basil, ground, one teaspoon
- Black pepper, one teaspoon

- Tomatoes, eight large sliced in half
- Paprika, ground, one teaspoon
- Extra virgin olive oil, two tablespoons
- Parsley, two tablespoons, chopped
- Mozzarella cheese, sliced eight slices
- Lemon juice, four tablespoons

Instructions:

Drizzle the lemon juice on the inside parts of the sliced tomatoes and then sprinkles them with basil and black pepper. Set two tomato halves on each of four serving plates. Place one slice of cheese on each tomato half and then sprinkle on the paprika and the parsley. Sprinkle the olive oil over the tomatoes and serve.

Peppers Stuffed With Chicken Salad

Prep thirty min/serves six/calories 116
Gluten-free

Ingredients:

- Black pepper, one-half teaspoon
- Chicken breast, cooked and cubed, two cups
- Red onion, diced, one-fourth cup
- Greek yogurt, plain, two-thirds cup
- Cherry tomatoes, one pint cut into quarters
- Dijon mustard, two tablespoons
- Rice vinegar, two tablespoons
- Cucumber, one-half peeled and diced
- Parsley, fresh chopped, one-third cup
- Celery, sliced thinly, four stalks
- Green bell peppers, three, seeded and cut in half around the middle

Instructions:

In a large-sized mixing bowl, blend together the parsley, black pepper, yogurt, mustard, and the rice vinegar and let this set for thirty minutes so the flavors will blend. Then add in the chicken, celery, tomatoes, cucumbers, and onion and blend well. Spoon this mixture evenly into the bell pepper halves.

Grilled Chicory Rolls

Prep five min/cook ten min/serves eight/calories 79
Gluten-free and vegan

Ingredients:

- Parsley, dried, two tablespoons
- Tomato, one large
- Black pepper, one teaspoon
- Extra virgin olive oil, two tablespoons
- Thyme, one-half teaspoon
- Red chicory, eight leaves
- Red onion, sliced thin, eight slices

Instructions:

Wash and dry the chicory leaves. Slice the tomato into eight thin slices and sprinkle them with the thyme. Brush the olive oil on the chicory leaves and then season them with the black pepper and the parsley. Lay one slice of tomato and one slice of onion on each chicory leaf and roll each leaf and serve.

Lime Parsley Slaw Salad

Prep ten min/serves five/calories 119
Gluten-free and vegan

Ingredients:

- Avocados, two
- Parsley, fresh, chopped finely, one cup
- Green cabbage, one-half head shredded
- Red onion, diced, one-half cup
- Turmeric, one teaspoon
- Purple cabbage, one-half head shredded
- Garlic, minced, two tablespoons
- Rosemary, one teaspoon
- Paprika, one teaspoon
- Lime juice, two tablespoons
- Water, one-quarter of one cup

Instructions:

Blend the chopped parsley into the minced garlic. Peel the avocados and mash the pulp in a larger mixing bowl. Blend in the water and the lime juice with the parsley garlic mix until the avocado mix is smooth and creamy. Pour in the shredded purple and green cabbages and the red onion and mix everything completely. Set the slaw in the refrigerator for one hour before you serve it.

Zucchini Noodles With Avocado Sauce

Prep ten min/serves two/calories 313
Gluten-free and vegan

Ingredients:

- Avocado, one
- Water, one-third of one cup
- Parsley, freshly chopped, one and one fourth cup
- Cherry tomatoes, twelve sliced in thirds
- Turmeric, one teaspoon
- Capers, one tablespoon
- Walnuts, chopped finely, four tablespoons
- Lemon juice, two tablespoons
- Frozen zucchini noodles thawed and dried, one pound

Instructions:

Put the pulp of the avocado into a blender with the parsley, walnuts, lemon juice, water, and turmeric and blend until all ingredients are smooth and creamy. Put the zucchini noodles into a large bowl and pour the blended sauce over them with the capers and tomatoes and toss everything gently but completely. Serve the salad immediately.

Onion and Pepper Pasta

Prep ten min/cook ten min/serves four/calories 135
Vegan

Ingredients:

- Whole wheat pasta, any shape, twelve ounces cooked
- Parsley, dried, one tablespoon
- Whole peeled tomatoes, one fourteen ounce can with juice
- Red bell pepper, one chopped
- Yellow bell peppers, two chopped
- Bird's eye chili, chopped, one-fourth teaspoon
- Black pepper, one teaspoon
- Turmeric, one teaspoon
- Extra virgin olive oil, three tablespoon
- Garlic, minced, one tablespoon
- Red onion, diced, one half cup

Instructions:

Fry the bird's eye chili, garlic, and onion in hot olive oil for five minutes. Blend in the peppers, turmeric, black pepper, and tomatoes and cook all of this together for fifteen minutes, stirring often. Add in the parsley and cook for one more minute. Then blend this mixture with the cooked pasta and serve.

Chicken Cutlets With Chicory Root

Prep fifteen min/cook twenty min/serves four/calories 300

Ingredients:

- Chicken cutlets, one pound
- Extra virgin olive oil, two tablespoons
- Chicory root, one pound chopped into two-inch pieces
- Broccoli, three cups steamed
- Black pepper, one teaspoon
- Turmeric, one tablespoon
- Vegetable broth, one cup
- Lemon juice, two tablespoons
- Garlic, minced, one tablespoon
- Rosemary, one teaspoon
- Buckwheat flour, one quarter cup

Instructions:

Stab a few holes in the chicory root pieces with a fork and microwave them for ten minutes on high. While the chicory root is cooking mix together the seasonings. Use this mixture to season the cutlets and then coat them with flour. Fry the cutlets for ten minutes on both sides using a medium-high heat and the oil. When the chicory root is soft, place them on a serving plate. Lay the cutlets on a serving plate on a paper towel to drain. Add the minced garlic to the skillet for thirty seconds. Add in the broth and lemon juice to the skillet and cook for three more minutes. Spoon this sauce over the chicken and serve.

Baked Fish With Vegetables

Prep five min/cook fifteen min/serves two/calories 180

Ingredients:

- DRY RUB
- Black pepper, one-fourth teaspoon
- Cinnamon, one-fourth teaspoon
- Sage, ground, one-fourth teaspoon
- Nutmeg, one-fourth teaspoon
- Onion powder, one-fourth teaspoon
- Parsley, dried, one teaspoon
- Garlic powder, one teaspoon
- Thyme, dried, one teaspoon

- FISH INGREDIENTS
- Whitefish fillets, two six-ounce skinless boneless
- Extra virgin olive oil, two tablespoons
- Red onion, three slices
- Capers, drained, two teaspoons
- Black olives, one half cup
- Artichokes, one cup

Instructions:

Heat your oven to 425. Mix together in a smaller bowl all of the ingredients for the dry rub, mixing them well in a small bowl. Tear off two sheets of aluminum foil just over one foot wide (about fourteen inches). Lay one fish fillet on each foil sheet. Sprinkle each fillet with one tablespoon of the dry rub. Place the artichokes, onions, olives, and capers over the fish fillets, and then sprinkle them with the remainder of the dry rub. Dribble the olive oil over the veggies. Wrap the foil packets closed by pulling all four sides to the top of the fish and rolling the pouch closed. Bake the pouches for fifteen minutes on a cookie sheet.

Sloppy Joes

Prep ten min/cook fifteen min/serves four/calories 240

Ingredients:

- Ground beef, one pound
- Whole grain or rye bread or rolls
- Tomato paste, one-fourth cup
- Worcestershire sauce, two teaspoons
- Thyme, one half teaspoon
- Red onion, one small diced finely
- Vegetable broth, low-sodium, three-fourths cup
- Bird's eye chili, finely diced, one-half teaspoon
- Celery, one stalk diced finely
- Garlic, minced, two tablespoons
- Black pepper, one teaspoon
- Turmeric, one teaspoon

Instructions:

Break the meat into small bits as you stir it around in a large skillet, cooking the ground beef until it is browned completely, for about ten minutes. When the meat is thoroughly cooked, stir in the onion, bird's eye chili, celery, and garlic and cook this mixture for five more minutes. Blend in the remainder of the list of ingredients and mix them together well. Turn the heat lower down and let the mix simmer for twenty minutes until it begins to thicken. Serve

the sloppy joes on rye or whole grain bread or
rolls.

Hamburger Kale Gratin

Prep ten min/cook twenty min/serves four/calories 350
Gluten-free

Ingredients:

- Ground beef, one pound
- Parsley, one tablespoon
- Kale, chopped, two cups
- Turmeric, one teaspoon
- Cheddar cheese, shredded, one cup
- Italian seasoning, one tablespoon
- Thyme, one half teaspoon
- Greek yogurt, low fat, four tablespoons
- Black pepper, one teaspoon
- Extra virgin olive oil, two tablespoons
- Olive oil spray oil

Instructions:

Heat the oven to 425. Fry the kale for five minutes in the hot oil. Use the spray oil to grease an eight-inch baking dish. Stir in the Greek yogurt into the kale and mix this together well and then pour this mixture into the greased baking pan. Cook the ground beef thoroughly and season it with the turmeric, thyme, and pepper, and then add this mix to the mix in the baking pan. Top with the shredded cheese and bake the casserole for twenty minutes.

<u>Cauliflower Fried Rice</u>

Prep five min/cook ten min/serves four/calories 132
Gluten-free and Vegan (use a soy sauce that is labeled gluten-free)

Ingredients:

- Tofu, firm, pressed and chopped into small pieces, four ounces
- Soy sauce, low-salt, two tablespoons
- Carrot, one-quarter cup chopped fine
- Extra virgin olive oil, two tablespoons
- Garlic, minced, two tablespoons
- Red bell pepper, one cleaned and diced finely
- Green onion, one-quarter of one cup
- Red onion, diced finely, one-fourth cup
- Sesame oil, toasted, one teaspoon
- Capers, two tablespoons
- Riced cauliflower, twelve ounces frozen or fresh
- Black olive, diced, one fourth cup

Instructions:

Fry the chopped carrots and the riced cauliflower in hot oil for five minutes while stirring them often. Into this mix, you will add the minced garlic capers, red onion, and the chopped green onions and stir them in well. Cook all of this mix for another five minutes.

Now stir in the small pieces of tofu and mix them in well with the other ingredients. Cook the mix with the tofu for five minutes, just to warm the tofu. Pour in the sesame oil and the soy sauce, stir these in quickly, and then serve sprinkled with the black olives.

Squash and Sweet Potato Patties

Prep fifteen min/cook ten min/serves two/calories 112
Gluten-free and vegan

Ingredients:

- Applesauce, unsweetened, one half cup
- Sweet potato, shredded, one cup
- Extra virgin olive oil, two tablespoons
- Squash, shredded, one cup
- Black pepper, one teaspoon
- Turmeric, ground, one-fourth teaspoon
- Kale, chopped, two cups
- Rosemary, dried, one-half teaspoon
- Garlic powder, one-half teaspoon
- Parsley, dried, one-fourth teaspoon

Instructions:

Blend together well the sweet potato, kale, squash, and applesauce together in a large mixing bowl. Stir in the turmeric, parsley, garlic powder, rosemary, and pepper and mix these seasonings thoroughly. While the oil is heating, divide the mixture in the bowl into four portions of equal size. When the olive oil is hot, set each portion in the skillet in the hot oil and push the portions down gently until they are one-half to one inch thick. Let the portions fry for five minutes before gently turning them over. Fry them on the other side for five minutes and serve them while they are hot.

**Veggie Nachos**

Prep fifteen min/serves six/calories 159
Vegan (use nutritional yeast instead of feta
cheese)

Ingredients:

- Parsley, fresh, one tablespoon minced
- Capers, two tablespoons
- Red onion, two tablespoons minced
- Black olives, two tablespoons chopped
- Feta cheese, one-fourth cup crumble
- Grape tomatoes, one-half cup, cut into quarters
- Red chicory, one cup chopped
- Pita chips, three cups whole grain
- Black pepper, one-fourth teaspoon
- Lemon juice, one tablespoon
- Extra virgin olive oil, two tablespoons
- Hummus, one-third cup prepared

Instructions:

Blend together the olive oil, black pepper, lemon juice, and hummus in a bowl. Spread the pita chips out on a serving platter. Use a spoon to drizzle three-fourths of the hummus mixture over the pita chips. Garnish the chips with the feta cheese or the tomatoes, red onion, nutritional yeast, chicory, capers, olives, and lettuce. Spoon the remainder of the hummus decoratively in the middle of the pita chips and garnish everything with the parsley.

Mediterranean Pasta

Prep five min/cook fifteen min/serves four to six/calories 267
Vegan (use nutritional yeast instead of parmesan cheese)

Ingredients:

- Parsley, fresh chopped, one-fourth cup
- Parmesan cheese, one-fourth cup
- Lemon juice, one-fourth cup
- Bird's eye chili, diced finely, one-half teaspoon
- Black pepper, one-half teaspoon
- Extra virgin olive oil, three tablespoons
- Black olives, six ounces whole pitted
- Artichoke hearts, one fourteen ounces can quartered
- Grape tomatoes, two cups
- Garlic, minced, three tablespoons
- Rosemary, one teaspoon
- Capers, two tablespoons
- Nutmeg, one teaspoon
- Angel hair pasta, whole wheat, six ounces cooked

Instructions:

Save half of the water that the pasta was cooked in. During the time the pasta is cooking, get the veggies ready by slicing the cherry tomatoes in half, chopping the artichokes, and slicing the olives. Use a large skillet for cooking the bird's eye chili, black pepper, garlic, and tomatoes for five minutes. Drop the drained pasta into the skillet and stir everything together rapidly. Mix in the olives, capers, lemon juice, and artichokes. If this pasta mix seems to be a bit dry, then use some of the saved pasta water to loosen it. When all of the ingredients are well mixed together, take the skillet from the heat and garnish with the parsley and the Parmesan cheese or the nutritional yeast.

Chicken Buckwheat Bowl

Prep thirty min/serves four/calories 432

Ingredients:

- Parsley, finely chop, two tablespoons
- Black pepper, one-half teaspoon
- Chicken breast, one pound cooked, boneless and skinless
- Feta cheese, one-fourth cup crumbled
- Celery, diced, one cup
- Walnuts, slivered, one-fourth cup
- Roasted red peppers, one seven-ounce jar rinsed
- Red onion, finely chopped, one-fourth cup
- Black olives, pitted and chopped, one-fourth cup
- Garlic, minced, one tablespoon
- Extra virgin olive oil, four tablespoons divided
- Buckwheat groats, two cups cooked
- Bird's eye chili, chopped, one-fourth teaspoon
- Turmeric, ground, one-fourth teaspoon
- Paprika, one teaspoon

Instructions:

Place the chicken breast on a plate and shred it or slice it very thin. Puree the turmeric, walnuts, paprika, garlic, bird's eye chili, and roasted peppers with two of the tablespoons of olive oil until it is smooth and creamy. In a large-sized mixing bowl, mix the buckwheat groats, olives, red onion, and the other two tablespoons of the olive oil very well. Spoon the mixture with the buckwheat groats into four bowls, making them evenly divided. Top the buckwheat with the chicken and the celery. Drizzle on the red pepper sauce. Garnish with parsley and feta.

Chickpea Celery and Cranberry Salad

Prep twenty min/serves four/calories 155
Gluten-free and vegan

Ingredients:

- Black pepper, one teaspoon
- Cherry tomatoes, red, one cup cut in halves
- Parsley, fresh, chopped, one-fourth cup
- Cherry tomatoes, yellow, one cup cut in halves
- Extra virgin olive oil, two tablespoons
- Cucumber, chopped, one cup
- Chickpeas, one cup drained and rinsed
- Red onion, sliced thin, one-half cup
- Lemon juice, two tablespoons
- Cranberries, one cup washed and sliced in halves
- Celery, chopped, one cup

Instructions:

Toss the cucumber, onion, celery, chickpeas, cranberries, and tomatoes in a medium-sized mixing bowl. In a separate smaller sized bowl, stir together well the lemon juice, olive oil, parsley, and pepper. Pour the bowl of wet ingredients over the bowl of dry ingredients and toss to mix them together gently but very well.

Salmon With Quinoa and Vegetables

Prep ten min/cook twenty min/serves four/calories 298

Ingredients:

- QUINOA
- Quinoa, one cup cooked per package directions
- Lemon zest, two tablespoons
- Celery, three-fourths cup diced
- Parsley, dried, two teaspoons
- Red onion, one-fourth cup diced fine
- Cherry tomatoes, one cup sliced in half

- SALMON
- Parsley, fresh chop, one fourth cup
- Black pepper, one fourth teaspoon
- Lemon, one cut into eight wedges
- Turmeric, one teaspoon
- Salmon fillets, four fillets of five ounces each
- Paprika, one half teaspoon
- Olive oil spray oil

Instructions:

Heat the oven to 400. Use an olive oil spray to grease a nine by thirteen inch baking dish. Lay the fish fillets in the baking dish. Mix the turmeric, pepper, and paprika in a small bowl and sprinkle on the fish. Lay the lemon wedges around the fish. Spoon the cooked quinoa around the fish. Use a medium-sized mixing bowl to toss together the lemon zest, tomatoes, parsley, onions, and celery and pour this mixture over the fish and the quinoa. Bake the fish for twenty minutes.

Kale Macaroni Cheese

Prep five min/cook twenty min/serves four/calories 344
Vegan (use nutritional yeast instead of feta cheese)

Ingredients:

- Parsley, chopped for garnish
- Black pepper, one-half teaspoon
- Italian seasoning, one-half teaspoon
- Almond milk, one cup
- Vegetable broth, one cup
- Elbow macaroni, whole wheat, two cups
- Feta cheese, one cup
- Kale, fresh, eight ounces
- Tomatoes, two fresh, diced
- Garlic, minced, two tablespoons
- Onion, one small finely diced
- Olive oil, two tablespoons

Instructions:

Cook the garlic and onions in the hot oil for five minutes. Stir in broth, macaroni, seasonings, milk, cheeses, kale, and tomatoes. Boil this mix while you are stirring frequently, then turn down the heat and simmer this mixture for fifteen minutes. Stir this often, about every two to three minutes, or the mixture will stick to the pan. Sprinkle the macaroni mixture with parsley and serve.

Sweet Potato and Black Bean Buckwheat Bowl

Prep thirty min/serves four/calories 334
Gluten-free and vegan

Ingredients:

- Sweet chili sauce, two tablespoons
- Black beans, one fifteen ounce can drain and rinse
- Kale, fresh, four cups chopped
- Sweet potato, one peeled and cubed
- Red onion, one fine chop
- Extra virgin olive oil, three tablespoons
- Water, one and one-half cups
- Capers, two tablespoons
- Garlic powder, one half teaspoon
- Long grain rice, three-fourths cup uncooked

Instructions:

Cook the rice in water with the garlic powder for twenty minutes. While the rice cooks fry the sweet potato cubes for eight minutes in the hot oil, stirring often. Mix in the kale, onion, and beans and cook for five more minutes. Stir in the sweet chili sauce and capers into the cooked rice and add this to the potato mix and serve.

Coconut Lemon Lentil Soup

Prep ten min/cook forty-five min/serves six/calories 161
Gluten-free and Vegan

Ingredients:

- Parsley, fresh, for garnish
- Red pepper flakes, crushed, one quarter teaspoon
- Extra virgin olive oil, two tablespoons
- Sea salt, one-half teaspoon
- Garlic, minced, three tablespoons
- Black pepper, one teaspoon
- Celery, three stalks chopped
- Coconut milk, full fat, one third cup
- Lemon juice, two tablespoons
- Tomato paste, one quarter cup
- Red lentils, two cups
- Water, four cups
- Vegetable broth, four cups
- Coriander, one-half teaspoon
- Turmeric, one and one-half teaspoon
- Capers, two tablespoons
- Paprika, one and one-half teaspoon
- Carrots, two chopped

Instructions:

Fry the onion in a large soup pot for five minutes in the hot oil. Add in the garlic and cook these for another three minutes. Mix in the coriander, turmeric, paprika, carrots, capers, and celery and fry this for five more minutes while stirring often. Then add in the lentils, water, tomato paste, and broth and mix well. Let this mix come to a boil and then cook it on simmer for forty to forty-five minutes so that the lentils are tender. Then mix in the coconut milk, salt, pepper, and lemon juice and stir. Top each serving with fresh parsley as desired.

Sesame Asian Soba Noodles

Prep fifteen min/cook fifteen min/serves four/calories 85
Gluten-free and Vegan

Ingredients:

- Soba noodles, twenty-four ounces
- Bird's eye chili, minced, two teaspoons
- Garlic, minced, two tablespoons
- Sea salt, one-half teaspoon
- Capers, one tablespoon
- Black pepper, one teaspoon
- Sesame oil, one tablespoon
- Rice vinegar, three tablespoons
- Parsley, fine chop, one-fourth cup packed

Instructions:

Cook the soba noodles. While they are cooking mix well in a large-size mixing bowl, the rice vinegar, sesame oil, black pepper, capers, sea salt, garlic, and chili until everything is blended together. When the noodles have completed cooking, drain them and put them into the large bowl and toss all of the mixture together well. Divide this into four serving bowls and sprinkle the parsley on top for garnish.

Avocado Mushroom and Chicory Root Salad

Prep ten min/cook twenty min/serves four/calories 370
Gluten-free and Vegan

Ingredients:

- Avocado, two ripe, peeled and sliced thin
- Rosemary, one teaspoon
- Chicory root, cooked and cooled, one cup chopped
- Lemon juice, one-fourth cup
- Portobello mushroom caps, four medium-sized
- Black pepper, one-half teaspoon
- Kale, chopped, one cup
- Red onion, one small, chopped finely
- Extra virgin olive oil, three tablespoons + one tablespoon
- Sea salt, one-half teaspoon and one half teaspoon

Instructions:

Heat the oven to 450. Brush both of the sides of the Portobello mushroom caps with the olive oil and sprinkle them with one of the one-half teaspoons of salt. Bake the caps for twenty minutes or until they are tender when they are stuck with a fork. While the caps are roasting, blend together the red onion, lemon juice, black pepper, rosemary, olive oil, and the other one-half teaspoon of salt. Use only half of this mixture to toss with the chicory root and the chopped kale in a medium-sized bowl until all is well mixed. Divide this veggie mixture over four serving plates. Lay the baked Portobello caps on top of this mixture on the plate. Top the mushroom caps with the slices of avocado. Serve the leftover of the dressing on the side for garnish.

Minestrone

Prep twenty min/cook one hour/serves eight/calories 220
Vegan

Ingredients:

- Arugula, freshly chopped, four cups
- Garlic, minced, three tablespoons
- Red onion, one small minced
- Whole wheat pasta shells, small, three-fourths cup
- Black pepper, one-half teaspoon
- Squash, one medium yellow, thinly sliced
- Zucchini, one medium, thinly sliced
- Sea salt, one teaspoon
- Thyme, one quarter teaspoon
- Turmeric, one teaspoon
- Basil, dried, one-half teaspoon
- Oregano, dried, one and one-half teaspoon
- Water, two cups
- Vegetable broth, four cups
- Parsley, dried, two tablespoons
- Carrots, one-half cup diced
- Diced tomatoes, one fourteen to fifteen ounce can
- Kidney beans, red, two fifteen ounce cans rinse and drain
- Cannellini beans, two fifteen ounce cans rinse and drain

- Extra virgin olive oil, three tablespoons
- Celery, one-half cup sliced thin

Instructions:

Cook the carrots, parsley, squash, celery, zucchini, garlic, and onion in the hot olive oil in a large soup pot for five minutes while stirring often. Pour in the salt, diced tomatoes, herbs, cannellini beans, water, kidney beans, pepper, and broth and stir well to blend all of the flavors together. Boil the mix, and then cook the soup at a simmer for thirty minutes. Drop in the arugula and pasta and simmer for thirty more minutes.

Chicken and Avocado Salad

Prep thirty-five min/cook one hour/serves four/calories 402
Gluten-free

Ingredients:

- CHICKEN
- Parsley, chopped, three tablespoons
- Oregano, dried, one tablespoon
- Turmeric, one teaspoon
- Extra virgin olive oil, three tablespoons
- Sea salt, one teaspoon
- Black pepper, one teaspoon
- Parsley, fresh, one tablespoon chopped
- Lemon juice, one-fourth cup
- Chicken breast, two pounds skinless and boneless

- SALAD
- Cherry tomatoes, one pint sliced
- Red chicory, two bunches chopped
- Extra virgin olive oil, one-third cup
- Mustard, whole grain, one tablespoon
- Chicken broth, three cups
- Avocados, two sliced thinly
- Capers, two tablespoons
- Red onion, one slice thinly
- Sea salt, one-half teaspoon
- Black pepper, one teaspoon
- Oregano, dried, one teaspoon
- Lemon juice, two tablespoons

- Buckwheat groats, one cup

Instructions:

Mix all ingredients listed under the heading 'chicken' together in a large bowl except for the chicken to make a marinade. Put the chicken in this marinade and refrigerate for one hour. Boil the broth and the buckwheat groats and then lower the heat and then simmer for forty minutes. Fry the chicken for fifteen minutes on each side. Mix the tomatoes, onion, and chicory leaves together and divide these into four servings. Add on the buckwheat groats, avocado slices, and chicken slices to each plate to serve.

Stuffed Eggplant

Prep ten min/cook forty min/serves four/calories 329
Gluten-free and Vegan

Ingredients:

- Parsley, fresh chop, three tablespoons to garnish
- Sea salt, one teaspoon
- Black pepper, one teaspoon
- Thyme, fresh chop, one teaspoon
- Turmeric, ground, one teaspoon
- Kale, two cups chop
- Garlic, minced, two tablespoons
- Extra virgin olive oil, three tablespoons divide
- Greek yogurt, plain, .5 cup
- Lemon juice, one tablespoon
- Lemon zest, one tablespoon
- Quinoa, cooked, two cups
- Mushrooms, button, one cup thinly sliced
- Red onion, one diced
- Eggplant, two medium-size cut in half

Instructions:

Heat the oven to 400. Use a spoon to scoop out one-third of the flesh of the eggplant and save it for another use. Use one and one-half tablespoons of the olive oil to coat the inside of the eggplant halves and place them on baking pan inside facing up. Use the remainder of the olive oil to cook the garlic, onions, mushrooms, kale, and quinoa for five minutes. Use lemon juice, turmeric, pepper, salt, and thyme to season this mix. Use the mix to fill the eggplant halves and bake them for twenty minutes. Sprinkle the eggplant halves with parsley and serve with sides of the yogurt for dipping.

Chicken and Buckwheat Salad

Prep fifteen minutes/cook 40 minutes/serves four/calories 264
Gluten-free

Ingredients:

- RED WINE VINAIGRETTE
- Honey, one teaspoon
- Lemon juice, two tablespoons
- Oregano, fresh, chop, one tablespoon
- Garlic, minced, two tablespoons
- Extra virgin olive oil, one-half cup
- Bird's eye chili, minced, one teaspoon
- Sea salt, one teaspoon
- Red wine vinegar, three tablespoons
- Black pepper, one teaspoon

- CHICKEN
- Chicken breast, one pound boneless and skinless cut into chunks
- Extra virgin olive oil, two tablespoons
- Balsamic vinegar, two tablespoons
- Parsley, chopped, one tablespoon
- Oregano, chopped, one tablespoon
- Paprika, one tablespoon
- Garlic, minced, two tablespoons
- Sea salt, one teaspoon
- Black pepper, one teaspoon
- Red potatoes, one pound cut in wedges
- Red bell pepper, one cleaned and diced small

- Buckwheat groats, two cups cooked
- Red chicory, one bunch chopped
- Feta, crumbled, one cup
- Red onion, cucumber, green and/or black olives, and tzatziki for serving

Instructions:

Heat the oven to 425. Mix together well the chicken, parsley, balsamic vinegar, salt, pepper, garlic, paprika, oregano, and one tablespoon of the olive oil. Lay the chicken in a thirteen by nine-inch baking dish and add in the bell peppers and potatoes. Bake this dish for forty-five minutes. Blend well all of the ingredients for the vinaigrette and set this to the side. Divide the red chicory and the buckwheat groats evenly between four serving bowls and add equal portions of the veggie and roast chicken mix. Drizzle the vinaigrette over the bowls and serve them with tzatziki, red onion, olives, and cucumber on the side.

Tuscany Style Vegetable Soup

Prep fifteen min/cook thirty min/serves eight/calories 225
Gluten-free and Vegan

Ingredients:

- Parsley, freshly chopped for garnish
- Red onion, one medium diced
- Zucchini, one medium peeled and chopped
- Extra virgin olive oil, three tablespoons
- Garlic, minced, two tablespoons
- Sea salt, one-half teaspoon
- Marjoram, one teaspoon
- Turmeric, one teaspoon
- Thyme, one-half teaspoon
- Vegetable broth, six cups
- Tomatoes, two large diced small
- Black pepper, one teaspoon
- Basil, ground, one tablespoon
- Kale, chopped, two cups
- Tomato paste, two tablespoons
- Celery, chopped, one-half cup
- Carrot, chopped, one-half cup

Instructions:

Fry the garlic and the red onion in the heated olive oil in a large soup pot for five minutes. Then add in the celery, carrots, and the zucchini and cook all of this for ten more minutes while stirring frequently. Mix in well the thyme, turmeric, tomatoes, marjoram, pepper, and salt and cook for five more minutes. Blend in the vegetable broth and the tomato paste and then let this boil. Cook the soup on simmer for fifteen minutes. Blend in the parsley and basil, and then take the pot off the stove and let the soup sit undisturbed for ten minutes. Garnish with fresh parsley and serve.

Buckwheat Vegetable Soup

Prep fifteen min/cook twenty min/serves eight/calories 165
Gluten-free and Vegan

Ingredients:

- Parsley, dried, two tablespoons
- Buckwheat groats, one cup, rinsed and uncooked
- Black pepper, one teaspoon
- Lemon juice, two tablespoons
- Sea salt, one teaspoon
- Garlic, minced, three tablespoons
- Red chicory, two cups shredded
- Lovage, chopped, one-half cup
- Broccoli florets, one cup
- Turmeric, one teaspoon
- Kale, one bunch, chopped with the stems removed
- Carrots, three peeled and diced
- Extra virgin olive oil, one tablespoon
- Red onion, one diced
- Vegetable broth, four cups
- Oregano, dried, one teaspoon
- Thyme, dried, one-half teaspoon
- Celery, three stalks diced

Instructions:

Use a Dutch oven or another large soup pot to warm the olive oil. Stir in the red onion, celery, and carrots and fry for five minutes. Stir in the oregano, turmeric, and thyme and mix well. Pour in the water and vegetable broth and bring this to a boil. Blend in the buckwheat groats and cook on simmer for fifteen minutes. Add in the cabbage, lovage, broccoli, and kale and cook for five more minutes, stirring occasionally. Blend in the salt, pepper, and lemon juice and serve.

Tropical Style Red Chicory Salad

Prep fifteen min/serves four/calories 155
Gluten-free and Vegan

Ingredients:

- Extra virgin olive oil, two tablespoons
- Black pepper, one-half teaspoon
- Pineapple, fresh, finely chopped, two cups
- Sea salt, one-half teaspoon
- Orange juice, two tablespoons
- Basil leaves, chopped, one-fourth cup firmly packed
- Red chicory root, cut into chunks, two cups
- Capers, two tablespoons

Instructions:

Heat your oven to 450. Cover the red chicory root with the olive oil. Bake the roots for ten minutes, turning over after five minutes. Allow the roots to cool. When the red chicory has cooled to room temperature, dice it into small bits, and then put the bits in a large-sized bowl. Add in the orange juice, basil, capers, pepper, salt, and pineapple and toss the ingredients gently but well to mix them together and coat all pieces well. You can eat it right away or save it in the refrigerator for no more than one day.

Pesto Pasta

Prep twenty min/cook twenty min/serves eight/calories 332
Vegan

Ingredients:

* Parsley, fresh, chopped, one-fourth cup packed
* Grape tomatoes, two cups cut into halves
* Pesto, vegan
* Lemon juice, one tablespoon
* Extra virgin olive oil, two tablespoons
* Green onions, four, trimmed and diced
* Green bell pepper, cleaned and sliced thin
* Zucchini, one medium, cut in half-inch-thick slices
* Kale, chopped, one cup
* Capers, two tablespoons
* Yellow squash, one medium cut into slices about one-half-inch thick
* Corn, frozen or canned and drained, two cups
* Whole wheat spaghetti, one pound

Instructions:

Use the directions on the package to cook the spaghetti. When the spaghetti is done cooking, drain the pasta well and let it cool completely. While the spaghetti is cooking, use a large size mixing bowl to blend together the capers,

zucchini, squash, onion, bell pepper, and corn
and toss them with the olive oil, pepper, and salt
until all of the ingredients are mixed together
well. Pour this mixture into a large skillet and
cook the ingredients on high heat, stirring
continuously, for about ten minutes until the
veggies are warm and have some charred spots.
In another bowl, mix together the lemon juice
with the pesto, and then mix this into the
cooked veggies. Toss in the cooled spaghetti
noodles, stir well to mix everything together,
and serve.

Chapter 9

Recipes For Dinner

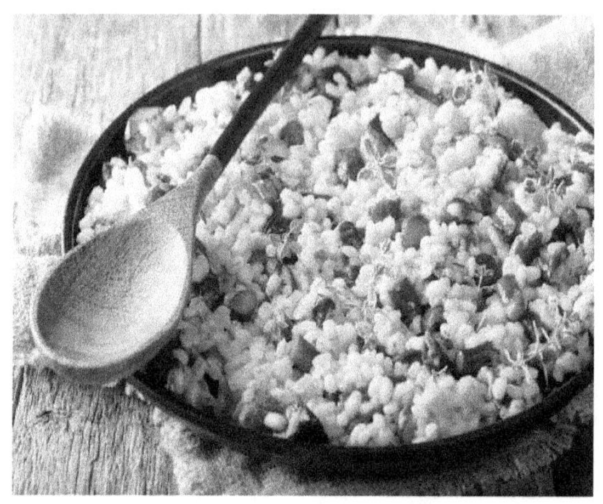

Buckwheat and Mushroom Risotto

Prep twenty minutes/cook thirty minutes/serves six/calories 297
Gluten-free and vegan

Ingredients:

- Black pepper, one teaspoon
- Sea salt, one half teaspoon
- Parsley, dried, one tablespoon

- Buckwheat groats, four cups
- Vegetable broth, two cups divided
- Mushrooms, button, one cup sliced thin
- Green bell pepper, one large, cleaned and minced
- Red onion, one small, well diced
- Capers, two teaspoons
- Garlic, minced, two tablespoons
- Marjoram, one teaspoon
- Extra virgin olive oil, two tablespoons

Instructions:

Fry the red onion, bell pepper, and garlic for five minutes in the olive oil. Pour into the skillet one cup of the vegetable broth and the mushrooms and cook these for five more minutes. Into this mixture, add the other cup of the vegetable broth and the buckwheat groats and cook all of this for ten minutes while stirring often. Pour in the capers, salt, pepper, and parsley and turn the heat under the pot to low. Simmer this mixture for fifteen minutes or until the buckwheat groats are completely cooked.

Halibut Chowder

Prep twenty min/cook one hour ten min/serves eight/calories 262
Gluten-free

Ingredients:

- Black pepper, one teaspoon
- Extra virgin olive oil, one-fourth cup
- Thyme, dried, one-fourth teaspoon
- Tomato juice, one cup
- Turmeric, one teaspoon
- Basil, dried, one-half teaspoon
- Sea salt, one-half teaspoon
- Parsley, fresh, chopped, two tablespoons
- Whole peeled tomatoes, two sixteen-ounce cans mashed with the juice
- Garlic, minced, three tablespoons
- Celery, three stalks chopped
- Red onion, one medium peeled and chopped
- Apple juice, one-half cup
- Red bell pepper, one cleaned and chopped
- Halibut steaks cut into cubes, three pounds

Instructions:

Cook the celery, garlic, onion, and peppers in hot oil in a large soup pot for five minutes. Blend in the apple juice, herbs, mashed tomatoes, and tomato juice and stir everything together well. Simmer this mix for thirty minutes. Drop the halibut pieces into the soup while stirring slowly. Add the pepper and salt and simmer for thirty more minutes.

Lamb Stew

Prep twenty-five min/cook one hour ten min/serves six/calories 389
Gluten-free

Ingredients:

- Red wine, one-half cup
- Parsley, fresh chop, three tablespoons
- Turmeric, one teaspoon
- Red bell pepper, one, seeded and chopped
- Sea salt, one teaspoon
- Zucchini, two small, peel, and slice
- Lamb shoulder, boneless, two pounds cubed
- Green beans, fresh, two cups trimmed
- Potatoes, four, peeled and cubed
- Oregano, dried, one teaspoon
- Extra virgin olive oil, two tablespoons
- Kale, chopped, one cup
- Tomatoes, peeled and chopped, four cups
- Chicken broth, one-half cup
- Garlic, minced, three tablespoons
- Black pepper, one teaspoon

Instructions:

Sprinkle the salt and pepper on the lamb and cook it with the minced garlic in the hot oil in a large soup pot for five minutes. Mix in the broth and red wine and let this boil. Lower the heat and put in the oregano and tomatoes, stir everything together well and simmer for forty-five minutes. Bring the soup back to an almost boil and stir in the red pepper, zucchini, green beans, and potatoes and cook for twenty more minutes while stirring often. Sprinkle the parsley on the soup to serve.

Celery and Smoked Sausage Soup

Prep twenty min/cook one hour ten min/serves eight/calories 404
Gluten-free

Ingredients:

- Thyme, crushed, one-half teaspoon
- Sea salt, one-half teaspoon
- Red onion, one chopped
- Extra virgin olive oil, one tablespoon
- Chicken broth, one cup
- Crushed tomatoes, one twenty-eight ounce can,
- Tomato sauce, one eight-ounce can
- Red beans, one fifteen ounce can with liquid
- Water, three cups
- Smoked sausage, one pound sliced
- Buckwheat groats, one-third cup uncooked
- Celery, six stalks diced
- Carrots, three diced
- Red chicory, one bunch, chopped

Instructions:

Fry the red onion in the hot oil for five minutes. Stir the water and sausage into the pot. Add in the celery, carrots, crushed tomatoes, tomato sauce, beans, buckwheat groats, and chicory and mix everything together well. Mix in the bay leaf, salt, thyme, and broth. Boil all of this for one minute, and then lower the heat and let the soup simmer for one hour.

Baked Cod With Maple Mustard Sauce

Prep ten min/cook fifteen min/serves two/calories 211
Gluten-free

Ingredients:

- Cod, two fillets, four ounces each fillet
- Lemon juice, one teaspoon
- Dijon mustard, three tablespoons
- Poppyseed, one teaspoon
- Red onion, chopped, one-fourth cup
- Sea salt, one-half teaspoon
- Black pepper, one teaspoon
- Turmeric, one teaspoon
- Mustard powder, one-fourth teaspoon
- Maple syrup, two tablespoons (can substitute honey)
- Garlic powder, one-half teaspoon
- Extra virgin olive oil, one tablespoon

Instructions:

Heat the oven to 400 degrees. Mix the mustard, maple syrup, turmeric, salt, pepper, garlic powder, poppy seed, oil, and mustard powder and set this off to the side to let the flavors blend together. Spread two tablespoons of this mix on the top of each fish fillet. Sprinkle the chopped red onion on the top of the fish. Bake the fish for fifteen minutes. Drizzle the lemon juice on the fish fillets before serving.

Philly Cheese Steak

Prep ten min/cook ten min/serves four/calories 350
General Diet

Ingredients:

- Extra virgin olive oil, one tablespoon
- Sirloin steak, one pound
- Black pepper, one teaspoon
- Red onion, one small sliced paper-thin
- Provolone cheese, low fat, four slices
- Green bell pepper, one medium cleaned and sliced thinly
- Parsley, dried, one tablespoon
- Whole grain bread, four slices, or four sub rolls

Instructions:

Slice the steak into strips that are very thin, about one-eighth of an inch thick, and then season the strips with the pepper. Fry the strips of the steak in hot oil until they are browned, between five and ten minutes. Drain the steak on a few paper towels, and then add in the green peppers and the onion and fry these for five minutes. Put one slice of cheese on each slice of whole-grain bread or sub roll and top the cheese with the steak slices and the onion and green pepper mixture, then sprinkle on the dried parsley and serve.

Thai Soup

Prep ten min/cook fifteen min/serves four/calories 339
Gluten-free and Vegan

Ingredients:

- Bell pepper, red, one-half cut in julienne strips
- Parsley, one half of one cup chopped
- Tofu, firm, pressed and cubed, ten ounces
- Vegetable broth, two cups
- Coconut milk, one fourteen ounce can
- Garlic, minced, two tablespoons
- Bird's eye chili, minced, one teaspoon
- Soy sauce, two tablespoons
- Turmeric, ground, one teaspoon
- Ginger, ground, one tablespoon
- Lime juice, two tablespoons
- Mushrooms, button, one-half cup
- Red onion, one-half cut in julienne strips
- Tamari, one tablespoon

Instructions:

Set on the stove, a large soup pot, and make the heat to a medium-high level. Pour in the vegetables broth and the coconut milk and stir them together well. Stir in the ground ginger, mushrooms, turmeric, garlic, bird's eye chili, red bell pepper, and onion and mix these ingredients all together well. Right when the liquid in the pot begins to boil, keep stirring the soup often and let the soup cook for five minutes. Now add in the tofu and let the mixture cook for another five minutes. Take the pot of soup off of the heat and stir in well the soy sauce, lime juice, parsley, and the tamari. Mix everything together well and then serve the soup.

Salmon With Buckwheat and Vegetables

Prep ten min/cook twenty min/serves four/calories 222
Gluten-free

Ingredients:

- BUCKWHEAT
- Buckwheat groats, one cup cooked per the package directions
- Lemon zest, two tablespoons
- Celery, diced, three-fourths cup
- Parsley, dried, two teaspoons
- Red onion, one-fourth cup diced fine
- Cherry tomatoes, one cup sliced in half

- SALMON
- Parsley, fresh chop, one-fourth cup
- Black pepper, one-fourth teaspoon
- Lemon, one cut into eight wedges
- Turmeric, one teaspoon
- Salmon fillets, four fillets of five ounces each
- Paprika, one-half teaspoon
- Olive oil spray oil

Instructions:

Heat the oven to 400. With the olive oil spray grease a nine by thirteen inch baking dish. Lay the fish fillets in the baking dish. Mix the turmeric, pepper, and paprika in a small bowl and sprinkle this mixture on the fish. Lay the lemon wedges around the fish. Spoon the cooked buckwheat around the fish. In a medium-sized mixing bowl, toss together the lemon zest, tomatoes, basil, onions, and cucumber and pour this mixture over the fish and the quinoa in the dish for baking. Cover with foil and bake the dish for twenty minutes.

Korean Steak

Prep five min/cook ten min/serves
four/calories 350
Gluten-free

Ingredients:

- Turmeric, ground, one tablespoon
- Extra virgin olive oil, three tablespoons
- Sirloin steak, one pound sliced thinly
- Bird's eye chili, minced, one teaspoon
- Ginger, ground, one tablespoon
- Sesame seeds, two tablespoons
- Red onion, thinly sliced, one-half cup
- Red chicory, chopped, one-half cup
- Arugula, chopped, one-half cup

Instructions:

Season the pieces of steak with the turmeric and the ginger and then. Fry the red chicory, arugula, red onion, and bird's eye chili in the hot oil and stir repeatedly for two minutes. Then blend in the steak pieces and stir often while cooking the steak for eight minutes.

Ham Cheese and Caper Soufflé

Prep ten min/cook thirty min/serves four/calories 460
Gluten-free

Ingredients:

- Olive oil spray oil
- Ham, fully cooked and diced, two cups
- Garlic, minced, two tablespoons
- Kale, chopped, one cup
- Red onion, chopped, two tablespoons
- Black pepper, one teaspoon
- Greek yogurt, one half cup
- Capers, two tablespoons
- Cheddar cheese, low-fat, shredded, one cup
- Eggs, six large
- Extra virgin olive oil, two tablespoons

Instructions:

Heat the oven to 400. Use the olive oil spray to grease four six-ounce ramekins or other oven-safe dishes. Fry the garlic, kale, and the onion in the hot oil over medium heat for five minutes. Mix together the diced ham, capers, cheddar cheese, onion, and garlic in a large size mixing bowl. Beat together the yogurt with the eggs and pour this over the ham mixture in the bowl. Then add the fried garlic, kale, and onion to the bowl and mix everything together very well.

Divide the mixture among the oven dishes and
cook them for thirty minutes.

Zucchini Lasagna Rolls

Prep forty five min/cook thirty min/serves four/calories 324 per four rolls

Ingredients:

- Zucchini, three large trimmed
- Walnuts, chopped, one-fourth cup
- Black pepper, one-half teaspoon
- Bird's eye chili, minced, one-fourth teaspoon
- Garlic, minced, two teaspoons and two teaspoons
- Italian seasoning, one teaspoon
- Crushed tomatoes, two cups
- Sea salt, one-quarter teaspoon and one quarter teaspoon
- Extra virgin olive oil, four tablespoons divided
- Olive oil spray oil

Instructions:

Heat the oven to 425. With the spray oil grease a baking sheet. Cut full slices from each zucchini down the length about one-fourth inch thick. Use three tablespoons of the olive oil to coat the strips and then sprinkle on one-fourth teaspoon of the salt. Bake the zucchini strips for twenty-five minutes until the zucchini strips are soft. Lower the oven temp to 350. Mix the two teaspoons of the minced garlic, black pepper, bird's eye chili, Italian seasoning, and the tomatoes in a medium-size mixing bowl and mix everything together well. Pour the tomato mix into a greased nine by thirteen inch baking pan. Roll up each of the strips of zucchini and place them into the tomato mix in the pan. Bake these zucchini rolls for thirty minutes. Garnish them with the rest of the garlic and the chopped walnuts.

Kale Avocado and Black Bean Bowl

Prep twenty min/cook thirty min/serves four/calories 424

Ingredients:

- Kale, one bunch with the ribs removed and chopped into bite-sized pieces
- Bird's eye chili, minced, one quarter teaspoon
- Cherry tomatoes cut in half, one half cup
- Garlic, minced, two tablespoons
- Red onion, one chopped finely
- Black beans, two fifteen ounce cans drained and rinsed
- Cayenne pepper, one-fourth teaspoon
- Lime juice, one-fourth cup
- Parsley, chopped, one-half cup
- Salsa verde, mild, one-half cup
- Avocado, one, peeled, pitted, cut into big chunks
- Turmeric, one-half teaspoon
- Jalapeno, one-half, seeded and chopped finely
- Extra virgin olive oil, two tablespoons
- Sea salt, one-half teaspoon
- Buckwheat groats, one cup rinsed

Instructions:

Cook the buckwheat groats per the package instructions and then let them rest for fifteen minutes. Then stir the salt into the buckwheat groats and fluff them with a fork. While the rice is cooking, prepare the kale salad by blending together in a larger mixing bowl the turmeric, salt, olive oil, jalapeno, and the lime juice, and then add in the chopped kale. In another medium-size bowl mix together well the parsley, lime juice, salsa verde, and the chunks of the avocado. Warm the beans over a low heat in one tablespoon of the olive oil. Mix in the red onion and the garlic and cook these for three minutes, then stir in the bird's eye chili and cayenne pepper. Cook this mixture for seven to ten minutes. For serving, add the kale salad with the buckwheat groats and the bean mixture to bowls and add in some of the salsa verde avocado. Toss the chopped cherry tomatoes on top of each bowl for garnish.

Hasselback Caprese Chicken

Prep twenty five min/cook twenty-five min/serves four/calories 355
Gluten-free

Ingredients:

- Extra virgin olive oil, two tablespoons
- Chicken breast, two boneless and skinless
- Broccoli florets, eight cups
- Marjoram, one-half teaspoon
- Turmeric, one teaspoon
- Thyme, one-half teaspoon
- Pesto, prepared, one-fourth cup
- Black pepper, one-fourth teaspoon and one-fourth teaspoon
- Mozzarella, fresh, three ounces halved and sliced
- Tomato, one medium sliced
- Olive oil spray oil

Instructions:

Heat the oven to 375. Use the spray oil to grease a baking sheet. Cut evenly spaced lines across each chicken breast about one-half inch apart from one end of the breast to the other. Sprinkle the chicken breasts with the turmeric, black pepper, thyme, and marjoram. Fill the cut places on the chicken alternating with the cheese and tomato. Coat each of the chicken breasts with the pesto. Lay the chicken down one side of the baking sheet. Put the olive oil and the broccoli in a smaller bowl and toss well until the broccoli is completely coated. Put the broccoli on the empty side of the baking sheet, adding in any tomatoes that are leftover. Bake the chicken and the broccoli for thirty minutes.

Grape Tomatoes and Soba Noodles

Prep five min/cook ten min/serves two/calories 137
Gluten-free and Vegan

Ingredients:

- Soba noodles, sixteen ounces
- Extra virgin olive oil, one tablespoon
- Tarragon, one teaspoon
- Garlic, minced, two tablespoons
- Turmeric, one teaspoon
- Black pepper, one teaspoon
- Grape tomatoes, one cup cut in half
- Bird's eye chili, minced, one-fourth teaspoon
- Thyme, one-half teaspoon
- Parsley, fresh, chopped, one tablespoon

Instructions:

Fry the minced garlic for one minute in the hot oil. Add in the turmeric, tarragon, black pepper, bird's eye chili, thyme, and the tomatoes and mix well and then lower the heat. Simmer this mix for fifteen minutes. Stir in the parsley and the soba noodles, and then cook on a high heat the complete mixture for five minutes, stirring constantly.

Grilled Pork Tenderloin

Prep ten min/cook twenty min/serves four/calories 340
Gluten-free

Ingredients:

- Pork tenderloin, two pounds
- Black pepper, one teaspoon
- Extra virgin olive oil, one-fourth cup
- Bird's eye chili, minced, one teaspoon
- Apple cider vinegar, one-half cup
- Dijon mustard, three tablespoons
- Garlic, minced, two tablespoons

Instructions:

Use a large size mixing bowl to mix together the mustard, apple cider vinegar, bird's eye chili, garlic, black pepper, and olive oil until all of the ingredients are well blended. Place the pork tenderloin into this mixture and let it set in the refrigerator overnight. The next day take the tenderloin out of the marinade and let it come to room temperature before grilling. Throw the marinade away. Grill the pork tenderloin for ten minutes on each side or until a meat thermometer reads 160 degrees in the tenderloin. Allow the tenderloin to stand for ten minutes before slicing it. Serve the slices of pork tenderloin with the Dijon mustard.

<u>Tofu in Tomatoes</u>

Prep five min/cook twenty min/serves two/calories 284
Gluten-free and Vegan

Ingredients:

- Thyme, one quarter teaspoon
- Turmeric, one teaspoon
- Tomatoes, one fifteen ounce can diced
- Black pepper, one teaspoon
- Extra virgin olive oil, one tablespoon
- Rosemary, one teaspoon
- Bird's eye chili, minced, one teaspoon
- Oregano, one teaspoon
- Parsley, dried, one teaspoon
- Garlic, minced, two tablespoons
- Tofu, one block medium, unpressed, cut into rounds one-half-inch thick

Instructions:

Fry the minced garlic for two minutes in the hot olive oil. Blend in the turmeric, rosemary, bird's eye chili, thyme, oregano, pepper, and the tomatoes, mixing these ingredients together well. After they are well-mixed, turn down the heat under the skillet so that the mixture can simmer. Let the mix simmer for five minutes. Lay the rounded slices of tofu into the tomato mixture and then let the mix simmer undisturbed for fifteen minutes, or until the sauce is somewhat thick and the tofu has begun to get soft. Sprinkle the dried parsley over the top for a garnish.

Greek Style Spaghetti Squash

Prep forty min/cook thirty min/serves two/calories 272
Gluten-free and vegan

Ingredients:

- Extra virgin olive oil, two tablespoons
- Thyme, dried, one-half teaspoon
- Red onion, one-fourth cup sliced thinly
- Marjoram, dried, one teaspoon
- Cherry tomatoes, eight, each cut in three slices
- Arugula, fresh, chopped, one cup
- Chickpeas, one-third of one cup, drained and rinsed
- Nutritional yeast, two tablespoons
- Rosemary, dried, one teaspoon
- Spaghetti squash, one large
- Garlic, minced, one tablespoon
- Turmeric, one teaspoon
- Capers, two tablespoons
- Olive oil spray oil

Instructions:

Heat the oven to 400. Rinse off and dry the outside of the spaghetti squash and then cut it in half from one end to the other end. Scoop out the seeds and discard them. Lightly oil the insides of the squash with one tablespoon of the olive oil. Completely cover a baking pan with the spray lightly coated. Lay the spaghetti squash on the cookie sheet with the inside facing down. Use a dinner fork to stab three or four sets of holes into the skin of the squash to allow the steam and heat to escape during cooking, and then bake the squash for thirty minutes. When the squash is done, use the tines of a fork to scrape the cooked flesh out of the spaghetti squash; pulling it out with a fork will make it look like strands of spaghetti. Put the stringed squash in a bowl and set it off to the side. Fry the onion, capers, and the garlic in the last tablespoon of the olive oil for five minutes while stirring occasionally. Then blend in the turmeric, rosemary, marjoram, thyme, tomatoes, and chickpeas and cook this mix for five more minutes. Mix in the arugula and the spaghetti squash and stir constantly while you cook this for five more minutes. Sprinkle the nutritional yeast on top and serve while the dish is hot.

Creamy Curry Noodles With Kale

Prep ten min/cook ten min/serves four/calories 205
Gluten-free and Vegan

Ingredients:

- NOODLE BOWL
- Red bell pepper, one cleaned and diced
- Carrots, two, peeled and cut in julienne strips
- Cauliflower, one-half of one head chopped small
- Parsley, fresh, chopped small, one-half cup
- Celery, two stalks chopped
- Kale, two cups packed
- Zucchini noodles, one sixteen ounce pack
- Celery, two, cut into chunks
- Boiling water, two cups

- CREAMY CURRY SAUCE
- Water, one-quarter cup
- Apple cider vinegar, two tablespoons
- Tahini, one-quarter cup
- Extra virgin olive oil, two tablespoons
- Ginger, ground, one quarter teaspoon
- Black pepper, one-half teaspoon
- Coriander, ground, one and one-half teaspoons
- Turmeric, ground, one teaspoon

- Curry powder, two teaspoons

Instructions:

Cover the zucchini noodles with the two cups of boiling water in a large size mixing bowl. Set this bowl off to the side to let the noodles steam. After five minutes, drain the water off and then put the hot noodles back into the bowl. After prepping the veggies toss the celery, bell pepper, carrots, parsley, and cauliflower into the noodles. Lay the kale leaves out onto four individual serving plates. Put together all of the ingredients for the Curry Sauce and mix it well in a medium-size mixing bowl. Pour over the ingredients the creamy sauce in the large mixing bowl with the noodles and toss everything together gently but very well. Divide the noodle mix over the kale leaves on the plates and serve.

Portobello Mushroom and Chicory Tacos

Prep twenty min/cook ten min/yields six tacos/calories 405 for two tacos
Gluten-free and Vegan

Ingredients:

- GUACAMOLE
- Lime juice, two tablespoons
- Parsley, chopped fine, one tablespoon
- Avocado, two medium-sized
- Tomatoes, chopped fine, two tablespoons
- Bird's eye chili, minced, one teaspoon
- Red onion, chopped fine, two tablespoons

- TACOS
- Portobello mushrooms, one pound
- Turmeric, ground, one teaspoon
- Onion powder, one teaspoon
- Red chicory leaves, six
- Extra virgin olive oil, three tablespoons divided
- Harissa, mild or spicy, one-quarter cup

Instructions:

Clean off the gills and stems from the Portobello mushrooms if you have not purchased just the caps. Rinse off the mushroom caps and pat them dry. In a smaller bowl, blend together the onion powder, turmeric, harissa, and one and one-half tablespoons of the olive oil until all ingredients are creamy and smooth. Completely cover the underside of each of the mushroom caps with this mixture, making sure to cover the edges too. Let them sit and marinate for fifteen minutes. Mix up the ingredients for the guacamole while you are letting the mushrooms marinade. After wiping off the avocados cut them in half and use a spoon to scoop out the flesh. Put the flesh into a medium-sized bowl and stir in the bird's eye chili, lime juice, parsley, red onion, and the chopped tomatoes. Rinse and dry the leaves of the red chicory. When the mushrooms have finished marinating, put the leftover of the olive oil in a skillet and let it get hot over a medium-high heat. Put the mushroom caps in the hot oil and fry them for three minutes on each side. Take the mushrooms out of the oil and lay them on a plate you have placed paper towels on to drain. Leave the mushrooms to rest for five minutes before you slice them. Lay a few slices of the mushroom cap in a collard leaf. Top the slices with the guacamole and the harissa and enjoy.

Egg Roll in a Bowl

Prep five min/cook fifteen min/serves two/calories 178
Gluten-free and Vegan

Ingredients:

- Carrots, two shredded to make one cup
- Extra virgin olive oil, one tablespoon
- Sesame seeds, one-quarter cup for garnish
- Black pepper, one teaspoon
- Sesame oil, one teaspoon
- Red onion, one-half sliced thin
- Mushrooms, one cup sliced
- Tamari, two tablespoons
- Red chicory, four cups shredded
- Celery, two stalks minced
- Green onions, chopped, one-half cup for garnish

Instructions:

Fry the carrots, celery, and onions in hot oil for five minutes. Pour in the tamari, pepper, mushrooms, and shredded red chicory. Stir all these ingredients together well. Drop the heat to low under the skillet and let the mix simmer for fifteen minutes. Stir in the sesame oil for one minute and then take the pan off of the heat. Serve with the sesame seeds and the chopped green onions for garnish.

Herbed Grilled Cod

Prep ten min/cook twenty min/serves four/calories 275
Gluten-free

Ingredients:

- Extra virgin olive oil, two to four tablespoons
- Cod fillets, eight pieces
- Peppercorns, whole, one teaspoon
- Turmeric, one teaspoon
- Black pepper, one teaspoon
- Rosemary, dried, one tablespoon
- Dried fennel seeds, one teaspoon
- Garlic, minced, two teaspoons
- Thyme, dried, one tablespoon

Instructions:

Put the fennel seeds, rosemary, peppercorns, thyme, garlic, turmeric, and the black pepper into a small bowl and mix them all together well. Coat both sides of the cod fillets with the olive oil. Press the cod fillets gently but deeply into the bowl of seasonings to coat both sides very well. Put the fillets on a plate and cover them and let the fish chill in the refrigerator for two hours. Cook the cod fillets under the broiler, five inches below the coils, or grill them on an outdoor grill for eight minutes on each side. Serve with a salad of fresh greens.

Indian Roasted Vegetables

Prep ten min/cook twenty min/serves four/calories 156
Gluten-free and Vegan

Ingredients:

- MASALA SEASONING
- Turmeric, one teaspoon
- Garlic, minced, one tablespoon
- Black pepper, one teaspoon
- Tomato puree, one-half cup
- Extra virgin olive oil, two tablespoons
- Chili powder, ground, one-half teaspoon
- Ginger, ground, two teaspoons
- Garam masala, one-fourth teaspoon
- Olive oil spray oil

- VEGGIES
- Green beans, three-fourths cup
- Celery, three stalks cut into chunks
- Red chicory root, cut into chunks, one cup
- Mushrooms, sliced, one-half cup
- Cauliflower, one cup in small pieces

- GARNISH
- Red onion, diced, one-half cup
- Parsley, chopped, one-fourth cup

Instructions:

Heat the oven to 400 and set the rack in the oven in the middle. Use olive oil spray to spray oil a baking sheet. If the veggies have not been chopped, then chop them now. In a medium-sized mixing bowl, blend well together with the garlic, ginger, garam masala, chili powder, pepper, and the tomato puree until all of the ingredients are mixed well together, then blend in the olive oil. Put the chopped veggies into this mix and stir them around until all of the veggies are covered well with the tomato mixture. Lay the veggies out in a single layer on the coated baking sheet. Roast the veggies for twenty to thirty minutes or until the veggies are cooked the way you like them.

Shrimp With Lemon and Garlic Pasta

Prep ten min/cook twenty min/serves four/calories 464
General diet

Ingredients:

- Jumbo shrimp, one pound peeled and deveined
- Zucchini, two cups sliced thin
- Celery, three stalks cut into strips
- Grape tomatoes, one cup cut in halves
- Parsley, chopped, one tablespoon
- Capers, two tablespoons
- Garlic, minced, one tablespoon
- Whole grain pasta any style, eight ounces
- Bird's eye chili, minced, one-fourth teaspoon
- Extra virgin olive oil, three tablespoons
- Lemon zest, one tablespoon
- Black pepper, one teaspoon
- Lemon juice, two tablespoons

Instructions:

Cook the pasta per the package directions. While the pasta is cooking, cook the celery strips and zucchini with the black pepper for five minutes. Mix in the tomatoes and cook for three more minutes. Stir in the shrimp, bird's eye chili, parsley, and garlic and mix well. Cook this mixture for five minutes, stirring often, until the shrimp is done. The shrimp will turn a lovely pink when it is completely cooked. Stir the shrimp mix into the drained cooked pasta and mix well.

Feta Chicken Pasta

Prep five min/cook thirty min/serves four/calories 390
General diet

Ingredients:

- Parsley, fresh, finely chopped for garnish
- Extra virgin olive oil, two tablespoons
- Diced tomatoes, two fourteen ounce cans with spices
- Water, two cups
- Feta cheese, four ounces divided
- Black pepper, one-half teaspoon
- Capers, two tablespoons
- Whole wheat fettuccine, one pound
- Turmeric, one teaspoon
- Kale, chopped, one cup
- Chicken breast, two pounds cooked skinless and boneless, cut into chunks

Instructions:

Cook the chunks of the chicken breast in hot olive oil in a large pot for ten minutes, stirring often to cook all sides of chicken. Sprinkle on half of the pepper while stirring. Pour in the kale, turmeric, water, capers, and the diced tomatoes. Break the pasta in half and stir the pieces in, cooking them for ten minutes. Stir in one-half of the feta cheese and cook this mixture for five more minutes. Garnish with the fresh parsley and the other half of the feta cheese.

Cauliflower Pie

Prep thirty min/cook thirty min/serves four/calories 400
Gluten-free and Vegan

Ingredients:

- Balsamic vinegar, one-fourth cup
- Vegetable broth, one cup
- Garlic, minced, three tablespoons
- Mushrooms, diced small, one cup
- Black pepper, one teaspoon
- Tomato paste, one tablespoon
- Carrots, two medium-sized peeled and diced fine
- Thyme, dried, one teaspoon
- Dijon mustard, one tablespoon
- Nutritional yeast, three tablespoons
- Turmeric, ground, one teaspoon
- Nutmeg, ground, one teaspoon
- Cauliflower, one head broken into florets
- Red onion, one medium-sized diced finely
- Celery, one stalk washed and diced fine
- Extra virgin olive oil, two tablespoons

Instructions:

Heat the oven to 400. Cover the cauliflower with water in a medium-size saucepan, boil, and cook for eight to ten minutes or until the pieces of cauliflower are very tender. Drain the water off and put the cauliflower into a medium-sized bowl and set it off to the side. Heat the oil in a larger skillet and pour in the carrots, celery, and onion. Cook these for five minutes while stirring often. Put in the diced mushroom and fry these for another five minutes. Blend in the balsamic vinegar and the tomato paste. Cook for two minutes and then stir in the vegetable broth. Then simmer this mixture for ten minutes or at least until around half of the liquid has been absorbed. While this mix is cooking, mash the cooked cauliflower. When the cauliflower is well-mashed, add in the mustard, pepper, turmeric, thyme, nutmeg, and nutritional yeast. Pour the veggie mix into a square nine by nine-inch casserole dish and top with the mashed cauliflower mixture. Bake the casserole for twenty minutes.

Mixed Veggie Salad Bowl

Prep thirty min/cook twenty min/serves four/calories 313
Gluten-free and Vegan

Ingredients:

- SALAD
- Zucchini, one small
- Asparagus, one large bunch
- Walnuts, chopped, one-fourth cup
- Avocado, one cubed
- Arugula, fresh, two cups packed
- Red bell pepper, one medium
- Purple cabbage, shredded, one-half cup
- Extra virgin olive oil, two tablespoons
- Red chicory, shredded, one-half cup
- Celery, two stalks diced
- Capers, two tablespoons
- Parsley leaves, one-half cup packed

- VINAIGRETTE
- Extra virgin olive oil, three tablespoons
- Apple cider vinegar, two tablespoons
- Turmeric, one teaspoon
- Dijon mustard, two teaspoons
- Black pepper, one teaspoon

Instructions:

Heat the oven to 400. Peel off the skin of the zucchini and cut off the ends and then cut the zucchini into long strips and cut them into diagonal pieces about one-half-inch thick. Wash and clean the bell pepper and cut it into slices. Clean the asparagus. Chop the chicory and purple cabbage. Coat the veggies with the olive oil. Mix the veggies together well until all of the pieces are well coated with the oil and then lays them out in a flat layer on a baking pan. Cook the veggies for twenty minutes. While the veggies are baking mix together in a smaller bowl, all of the ingredients for the dressing. When the veggies are done baking, divide them evenly between four bowls, trying to get some of each veggie into each of the four bowls for a nice mixture, and then drizzle the mixed dressing over all of them and serve the salad immediately.

Beef and Blue Cheese Penne With Pesto

Prep ten min/cook twenty min/serves four/calories 432
General Diet

Ingredients:

- Gorgonzola cheese, one-fourth cup crumbled
- Beef tenderloin steaks, two, six ounces each
- Penne pasta, whole wheat, two cups cooked per package directions
- Black pepper, one-half teaspoon
- Walnuts, one-fourth cup chopped
- Pesto, already prepared, one-third cup
- Grape tomatoes, two cups halved
- Kale, fresh, six cups coarsely chopped

Instructions:

While the pasta is cooking broil the steaks five inches from the heating coils for seven minutes on each side. After the pasta is fully cooked, drain it and then pour the cooked pasta in a larger size bowl for mixing. Stir in the walnuts, pesto, tomatoes, and spinach and mix together well. Slice the steaks into quarter-inch thick slices and toss the slices with the pasta. Garnish with the cheese and serve.

Pepper Ricotta Primavera

Prep ten min/cook fifteen min/serves six/calories 232
Vegan

Ingredients:

- Fettucine, whole wheat, six ounces cooked and drained
- Almond milk, one-half cup
- Sweet red pepper, one medium cut in julienne strips
- Bird's eye chili, crushed, one-fourth teaspoon
- Ricotta cheese, part-skim, one cup
- Parsley, dried, one-fourth teaspoon
- Sweet yellow pepper, one medium cut in julienne strips
- Zucchini, one medium sliced thin
- Extra virgin olive oil, four tablespoons
- Garlic, minced, one tablespoon
- Oregano, dried, one-fourth teaspoon
- Turmeric, one teaspoon
- Peas, frozen, one cup thawed

Instructions:

Blend the almond milk and ricotta cheese and set this bowl off to the side. Fry the chopped bird's eye chili together with the minced garlic in the hot oil for two or three minutes or until they seem to be soft to the touch. Stir in the zucchini, sweet peppers, turmeric, oregano, peas, and parsley and cook all of this for five minutes while stirring occasionally. Pour the cheese mix over the fettuccine; add the vegetables from the skillet and toss everything together well.

Healthy Meatballs

Prep fifteen min/cook thirty min/serves four/calories 288
General Diet

Ingredients:

- Garlic, minced, two tablespoons
- Lime juice, one tablespoon
- Ground beef, two pounds
- Parsley, fresh chopped, one-fourth cup
- Turmeric, ground, one teaspoon
- Ginger, ground, one half teaspoon
- Olive oil spray oil

Instructions:

Heat the oven to 350. Use the spray oil to grease a baking sheet. Put all of the ingredients listed for the meatballs together in a larger bowl and mix them well. Form the mix into twelve meatballs of about an equal size. Set the meatballs on the baking sheet and bake them for thirty minutes. Serve the meatballs with a side vegetable or a tossed salad.

Beef and Avocado Burger

Prep five min/cook fifteen min/serves one/calories 295
Gluten-free

Ingredients:

- Black pepper, one-half teaspoon
- Ground beef, ninety percent lean, six ounces
- Turmeric, one teaspoon
- Mustard, yellow or whole grain, one teaspoon
- Avocado, one-quarter medium sliced thin
- Parsley, dried, one quarter teaspoon

Instructions:

Mix the pepper and parsley into the beef and then shape it into a patty about one-half inch thick. Fry the burger patty for five minutes on each side, or until it is cooked to your preference. Spoon the mustard on top and then add the slices of avocado.

Chapter 10

Recipes For Dessert

Desserts are allowed on the sirtfood diet. The beauty of the diet is that you are allowed to eat normal food that everyone else eats. Just make sure that the desserts that you eat are loaded with the sirtuin proteins that your body needs, so that will mean desserts made with blueberries, walnuts, strawberries, cocoa, and Medjool dates.

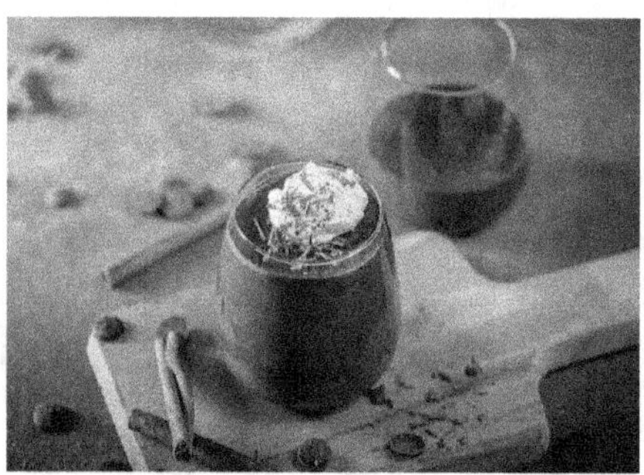

Chocolate Coffee Mousse

Prep four hours/cook fifteen min/serves eight/calories 242

Ingredients:

- Cocoa powder, two tablespoons
- Coconut yogurt, one and one-fourth cup
- Dark chocolate bar, chunked, three-fourths cup
- Cinnamon, ground, one teaspoon
- Maple syrup, two tablespoons
- Gelatin powder, one tablespoon
- Coffee, brewed, three-fourths cup
- Almond milk, one and one-fourth cup

Instructions:

Blend the coffee and the almond milk in a medium-size saucepan and sprinkle the gelatin on top of the liquid. Let the gelatin lay there for five minutes and then boil the mixture for two minutes. Take the pan from the heat and mix in the dark chocolate bar, cinnamon, and maple syrup. Keep stirring until the chocolate bar is completely melted. Pour the mousse into eight dessert dishes, dividing it evenly. Serve the mousse with one tablespoon of the coconut yogurt on top.

Chocolate Walnut Biscotti

Prep one hour/bake one hour/makes three to four dozen pieces/calories 132

Ingredients:

- Egg white, one beaten
- Walnuts, chopped, two cups
- Extra virgin olive oil, one cup
- Olive oil spray oil
- Cinnamon, one teaspoon
- Sea salt, one teaspoon
- Eggs, two
- Sugar, granulated, three-fourths cup
- Baking powder, one teaspoon
- Cocoa powder, unsweet, one-half cup
- Flour, all purpose, two and one-half cups
- Vanilla extract, one tablespoon

Instructions:

Heat the oven to 350. Use the olive oil spray to lightly coat two baking sheets. In a medium-size mixing bowl cream together the sugar, olive oil, vanilla extract, and eggs, until all of the ingredients are smooth. Use a large size bowl for the flour, baking powder, salt, cinnamon, and cocoa powder and blend these all together until they are well mixed. Put the mixture with the egg into the mixture of the flour and blend until all of the ingredients are well mixed, then put in the walnuts. Lay the dough out on the counter and pat it into a rough square shape, and then cut the dough across the middle both ways so that you have four squares that are about the same size. Roll each square into log shapes that are about one inch thick and coat them with the egg whites. Bake the logs, two on each baking sheet, for twenty-five minutes, and then let them sit undisturbed for ten minutes. Then gently slice the logs diagonally into cookie shapes that are about one-half inch think and return the cookies to the baking sheet. Bake them for another twenty minutes.

Dark Chocolate Bites

Prep ten min/makes fifteen/calories per bite 100

Ingredients:

* Water as needed
* Vanilla extract, one tablespoon
* Extra virgin olive oil, one tablespoon
* Turmeric, ground, one tablespoon
* Cocoa powder, one tablespoon
* Medjool dates, pits removed, one cup
* Dark chocolate chips, one-half cup
* Walnuts, chopped, one-half cup

Instructions:

Blend all of the ingredients listed together to form a soft ball of dough. Add in water as needed to make the dough pliable but not too wet. Pull the dough apart into lumps that will roll into balls that are bite-size. Place the chocolate balls into the refrigerator and let them chill for at least one hour before eating them

Strawberry Gelato

Prep thirty min/set twelve hours/calories 190 in one-half cups

Ingredients:

- Cornstarch, two tablespoons
- Strawberries, fresh, two pounds, cleaned and cut in quarters
- Heavy cream, three cups divided
- Sugar, granulated, one and one-half cups

Instructions:

Pour one-fourth of the heavy cream into a small size bowl and stir in the cornstarch until well blended. Set a medium-size saucepan on the stove and pour in the rest of the cream with the sugar. Set this over medium heat and stir often until the blend begins to simmer. Then stir in the cornstarch mixture and blend well and let this boil for two minutes. Put this mix into a bowl that is safe to put in the freezer and freeze it for ten hours.

Buckwheat Chocolate Chip Cookies

Prep ten min/cook eight min/makes thirty-six/calories per cookie 80

Ingredients:

- Mini dark chocolate chips, one-half cup
- Vanilla extract, one teaspoon
- Egg, large
- Granulated white sugar, one-fourth cup
- Sea salt, one-fourth teaspoon
- Cornstarch, one-half teaspoon
- Baking soda, one-half teaspoon
- Cinnamon, one teaspoon
- Extra virgin olive oil, one-half cup
- Rolled oats, old fashioned, one and one-half cups
- Buckwheat flour, one cup
- Brown sugar, packed, one-half cup
- Olive oil spray oil

Instructions:

Blend together the cornstarch, salt, baking soda, cinnamon, oats, and buckwheat flour in a medium-size mixing bowl. In another large-size bowl, cream together the sugar, olive oil, and brown sugar for three minutes until they are creamy and then stir in the vanilla extract and the egg. Slowly mix the flour mixture into the olive oil mixture, blending completely before adding more in. Gently fold in the chocolate chips and then put the bowl of cookie batter into the refrigerator for thirty minutes. Heat the oven to 350. After the dough has been in the refrigerator for at least thirty minutes, use the spray oil to cover a baking sheet and put the dough on it in tablespoons, leaving two inches between the balls of dough. Bake the cookies for eight to ten minutes.

Date Bars

Prep thirty min/bake thirty min/makes twelve bars/calories 238 per bar

Ingredients:

- Buckwheat groats, two cups
- Extra virgin olive oil, one-half cup
- Medjool dates, chopped, one cup
- Olive oil spray oil
- Orange juice, one-fourth cup
- Baking soda, one-half teaspoon
- Sugar, granulated, one-third cup
- Walnuts, chopped, one-half cup
- Rolled oats, one cup
- Egg, one
- Brown sugar, one cup packed
- Hot water, two tablespoons

Instructions:

Heat the oven to 350. Coat a nine by thirteen inch baking dish with the spray oil. In a small size mixing bowl, blend the walnuts, dates, orange juice, sugar, and hot water. Cream together in a larger size bowl the brown sugar, olive oil, and egg until they are creamy and smooth. Blend in the oats, flour, and baking soda. Put all of the dough except for one cup into the baking dish and press it into all of the corners. Drop the mixture with the dates on top of this dough and spread it around on the dough. The leftover dough will be dropped in small amounts on top of the date mix. Bake the cookie bars for thirty minutes and then cut them when they are completely cooled.

Buckwheat Double Chocolate Cookies

Prep twenty-five minutes/cook ten minutes/makes thirty/calories 118 per cookie

Ingredients:

- Vanilla extract/one teaspoon
- Extra virgin olive oil, six tablespoons
- Sea salt, one-half teaspoon
- Dark chocolate chips, one cup
- Granulated sugar, one-half cup
- Buckwheat flour, one-half cup
- Eggs, two
- Baking powder, three-fourths teaspoon
- Tapioca flour, two tablespoons
- Olive oil spray oil

Instructions:

Heat the oven to 350. Coat two baking sheets with the spray oil. In a medium-size saucepan and stir in the chocolate chips together with the olive oil and melt them over a low heat, stirring often. Take this mix off the stove and set it to the side. Whip together the salt, sugar, and eggs until they are smooth and creamy in a medium-size bowl. Then stir in the baking powder, tapioca flour, and the buckwheat flour. Then mix in the vanilla extract and the chocolate olive oil mixture and blend well. Drop heaping tablespoons of the batter on the baking sheets and bake the cookies for eight to twelve minutes.

Yogurt With Honey and Strawberries

Prep ten min/serves four/calories 176

Ingredients:

- Strawberries, sliced, one cup
- Walnuts, chopped, four tablespoons
- Honey, four teaspoons
- Greek yogurt, plain, three cups

Instructions:

Drop three-fourths of one cup of the Greek yogurt into each of one of four serving size dessert cups. Divide the sliced strawberries among the four dishes and arrange them on top of the yogurt. Drop one teaspoon of the honey and one tablespoon of almonds on top of each bowl of strawberries.

Maple Vanilla Baked Pears and Blueberries

Prep five min/cook twenty min/serves four/calories 198

Ingredients:

- Anjou pears, four
- Vanilla extract, one teaspoon
- Olive oil spray oil
- Blueberries, fresh or thawed frozen one cup
- Cinnamon, ground, one teaspoon
- Maple syrup, one-half cup

Instructions:

Heat your oven to 375. Use spray oil to cover lightly a baking sheet. Peel the pears and take out the pit, and then cut the pears in half the long way. Slice a bit out in the round part of each one so that they will stay still when you put them on the baking sheet. Lay the halves of pears on the baking sheet and cover the inside with the ground cinnamon. Then blend together the maple syrup and the vanilla extract and dribble half of it over the pear halves. Bake the pears for twenty-five minutes and then put each pear half into a dessert serving bowl. Cover each of the pear halves with one-fourth cup of blueberries and then dribble on the remainder of the maple and vanilla syrup.

Blueberry Walnut Crisp

Prep fifteen min/cook thirty min/serves nine/calories 222

Ingredients:

- TOPPING
- Extra virgin olive oil, one-fourth cup
- Nutmeg, ground, one-fourth teaspoon
- Cinnamon, ground, one teaspoon
- Walnuts, chopped, one-fourth cup
- Buckwheat flour, one-fourth cup
- Brown sugar, packed, one-third cup
- Rolled oats, old-fashioned, one-half cup

- FRUIT
- Granulated white sugar, two tablespoons
- Buckwheat flour, two tablespoons
- Lemon juice, two teaspoons
- Blueberries, frozen and thawed, two cups

Instructions:

Heat your oven to 350. Blend the lemon juice and blueberries together and pour them into an eight inch baking dish. Stir the white sugar and buckwheat flour into the blueberries carefully, so you don't crush the berries. In a medium-size mixing bowl, bend the nutmeg, cinnamon, walnuts, buckwheat flour, brown sugar, and the rolled oats until well mixed. Stir in the olive oil quickly to coat all of the ingredients and then drop spoonsful onto the blueberry mix. Bake the crumble for thirty minutes.

Chapter 11

Recipes For Sides And Snacks

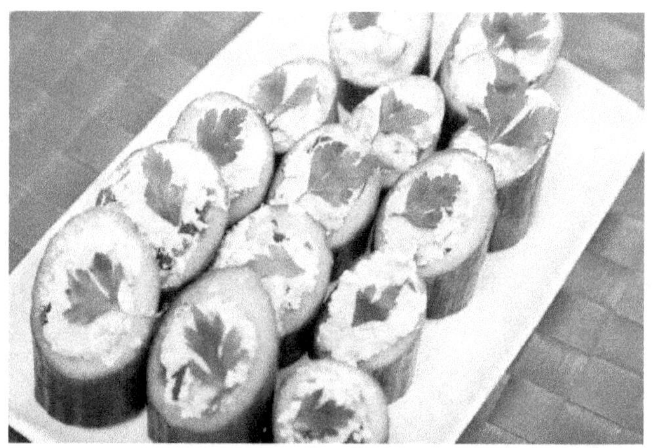

Cucumber Bites With Salmon and Avocado

Prep ten min/serves two/calories 246

Ingredients:

- Black pepper for garnish

- Smoked salmon, six ounces
- Lime juice, one-half tablespoon
- Red onion, chopped, one-fourth cup for garnish
- Cucumber, one medium-sized
- Avocado, one large, peel and remove pit

Instructions:

Peel the cucumber if and then slice it into slices that are about one-fourth inch thick, and then put the slices on a plate for serving. Cream together the lime juice and avocado until they are creamy and smooth. Put a teaspoon of the mashed avocado on each slice of cucumber, and then top the avocado with a slice of the smoked salmon. Use the onions and black pepper to garnish as you like.

Sprout Wraps

Prep fifteen min/serves two/calories 226 for three wraps

Ingredients:

- Red chicory leaves, six
- Extra virgin olive oil, one tablespoon
- Parsley, chopped, one-half cup
- Bean sprouts, one cup
- Carrots, grated, one-fourth cup
- Sea salt, one teaspoon
- Lemon juice, one tablespoon
- Celery, minced, one-fourth cup
- Red onion, minced, one-fourth
- Cucumber, one sliced thin
- Black pepper, one teaspoon

Instructions:

Lay out each of the red chicory leaves on a serving plate. Then evenly divide all of the listed ingredients between the red chicory leaves and then roll the leaves snugly around the ingredients.

Roasted Baby Eggplant

Prep twenty min/cook forty-five min/serves four/calories 44

Ingredients:

- TO COOK
- Baby eggplant, eight
- Black pepper, one teaspoon
- Sea salt, one teaspoon
- Rosemary, one teaspoon
- Extra virgin olive oil, two tablespoons

- FOR SERVING
- Black pepper, one teaspoon
- Ricotta cheese, low fat, one-half cup
- Sea salt, one teaspoon
- Turmeric, one teaspoon
- Extra virgin olive oil, two tablespoons

Instructions:

Heat the oven to 350. Rinse off the baby eggplant and dry them and then cut each one in half down the length. Set the baby eggplant on a baking pan with the inside facing up and then with the olive oil cover the insides and sprinkle on the rosemary, salt, and pepper. Bake the eggplant for forty-five minutes or until they become soft and start to turn slightly brown. Just before you serve the eggplant top, each one half with one teaspoon of the ricotta cheese and sprinkle that with the pepper, salt, and turmeric.

Roast Brussel Sprouts With Red Pepper and Garlic

Prep ten min/cook twenty min/serves four/calories 195

Ingredients:

- Bird's eye chili, crushed, one half teaspoon
- Black pepper, one teaspoon
- Garlic, minced, two tablespoons
- Turmeric, ground, one teaspoon
- Extra virgin olive oil, four tablespoons divided
- Brussel sprouts, two pounds

Instructions:

Heat the oven to 500. Trim off the bottom part from the Brussel sprouts and then put them into a medium-sized mixing bowl with the black pepper and two tablespoons of the olive oil. Toss the sprouts gently around until all of them are covered well. Spread the oily Brussel sprouts out onto a baking sheet and cover them over with a sheet of aluminum foil. Bake the sprouts for ten minutes and then take off the sheet of foil. Stir the Brussel sprouts around and then bake them for another ten minutes. While they are in the oven, put the remaining two tablespoons of the oil into a medium-sized skillet and fry the bird's eye chili and the minced garlic together for five minutes. When the

Brussel sprouts have finished cooking, mix them together with the fried garlic and red peppers, sprinkle the turmeric on the top, and serve.

Greek Yogurt Kale Dip

Prep ten min/bake thirty min/serves two/calories 230

Ingredients:

- Parmesan cheese, shredded, one-third cup
- Mozzarella cheese, shredded, two-thirds cup
- Feta cheese, crumbled, one cup
- Garlic, minced, two teaspoons
- Greek yogurt, plain, one and one-third cups
- Kale, chopped, two cups
- Turmeric, ground, one teaspoon
- Black pepper, one teaspoon
- Olive oil spray oil

Instructions:

Heat the oven to 350. Coat an eight by an eight-inch baking dish with the olive oil spray. Gently mix everything together in a medium-sized mixing bowl. Pour this mix into the coated baking dish and cook the dip for thirty minutes. Serve the dip hot with crackers, veggies, or chips.

Veggie Fritters

Prep ten min/cook fifteen min/serves four/calories 198

Ingredients:

- Extra virgin olive oil, three tablespoons for frying
- Garlic, minced, two tablespoons
- Red onions, two, minced
- Carrots, grated, one cup
- Celery, two stalks minced
- Cornstarch, one-fourth cup
- Egg, two
- Beets, two medium shredded
- Lemon juice, one-half teaspoon
- Turmeric, ground, one-half teaspoon
- Cumin, ground, two teaspoons
- Parsley, chopped, two tablespoons
- Black pepper, two teaspoons
- Coriander, ground, one-fourth teaspoon
- Cornstarch, four tablespoons

Instructions:

Fry the garlic and the onion in the hot olive oil for five minutes, and then pour everything from the skillet into a larger mixing bowl. Put in the pre-measured one-fourth cup of cornstarch, parsley, coriander, lemon juice, turmeric, cumin, celery, black pepper, parsley, beets, and carrots. Mix everything together well until all of the ingredients are blended completely. In another bowl, make a thick paste by beating the four tablespoons of cornstarch and the eggs together. Add this paste to the veggie mix and stir together until all of the ingredients are well mixed. Spoon the batter by tablespoons into the hot oil and fry for five minutes on each side.

Turkey Meatballs

Prep ten min/cook ten min/serves two/calories 302

Ingredients:

- Black pepper, one-fourth teaspoon
- Extra virgin olive oil, one tablespoon
- Sea salt, one-half teaspoon
- Red onion, grated, one-fourth cup
- Garlic powder, one-half teaspoon
- Turkey breast, ground, sixteen ounces
- Oregano, one teaspoon
- Feta cheese, one-half cup
- Parsley, dried, one-fourth teaspoon

Instructions:

Place the oven rack five inches below the broiler coils and then turn on the broiler in the oven. Mix all of the listed ingredients together well. Scoop two tablespoons of the mix out of the bowl and form it into the shape of a ball. Continue with all of the mix until you have made all of the meatballs. Then put all of the meatballs on a spray oiled baking sheet. Broil the meatballs for ten minutes.

Baby Red Potatoes With Spicy Olive Pesto

Prep ten min/cook thirty mon/serves six/calories 179

Ingredients:

- Sour cream, one-half cup
- Garlic, minced, two tablespoons
- Walnuts, chopped, one-half cup
- Extra virgin olive oil, six tablespoons divided
- Baby red potatoes, three pounds (about thirty-six)
- Bird's eye chili, minced, one teaspoon
- Red onion, minced, one-fourth cup
- Green olives, pimiento-stuffed, one and one-half cups
- Sea salt, two teaspoons

Instructions:

Heat the oven to 400. Rinse the potatoes well and let them dry, and then place them in a large size mixing bowl. Add in two tablespoons of the olive oil and the salt and mix well. Use spray oil to coat a baking sheet and put the potatoes on it, and then bake them for thirty minutes. Mix together the remainder of the olive oil with the bird's eye chili, walnuts, onion, garlic, and olives and blend until well mixed while the potatoes are baking. After the potatoes have cooled, slice a thin slice off the bottom of each one to allow them to sit upright. Cut two lines in the top of each potato, making them cross in the middle and gently squeeze the potatoes to make the cross open up. Use a teaspoon to fill each potato with the spicy pesto mix and garnish with sour cream if desired.

Roasted Chicory Root

Prep ten min/bake twenty min/serves one/calories 212

Ingredients:

- Black pepper, one-half teaspoon
- Extra virgin olive oil, two tablespoons
- Red chicory root cut into one-half inch pieces, two cups
- Garlic powder, one-half teaspoon
- Lemon juice, two teaspoons
- Red wine vinegar, two teaspoons
- Parsley, dried, one teaspoon
- Sea salt, one teaspoon
- Olive oil spray oil

Instructions:

Heat the oven to 425. Put the chunks of the chicory root onto a baking sheet that has been coated with the olive oil spray. Bake the chicory root for ten minutes, and then stir the pieces around and bake them for another ten minutes. Blend the remainder of the ingredients to mix together in a medium-size mixing bowl. After the chicory roots have baked the second time, put them into the bowl of mix and tosses them to coat the roots well. Bake the chicory root for another ten minutes, and then cool them and eat.

Roasted Root Veggies With Buttermilk Parsley Dip

Prep twenty min/cook twenty min/serves six/calories 265

Ingredients:

- BUTTERMILK PARSLEY DIP
- Sea salt, one-half teaspoon
- Buttermilk, six tablespoons
- Greek yogurt, low fat, eight ounces
- Honey, one teaspoon
- Garlic, minced, two tablespoons
- Parsley, minced, two tablespoons
- Lemon zest, one teaspoon

- ROOT VEGGIE CHIPS
- Turmeric, ground, one teaspoon
- Golden beet, one medium
- Red chicory root, one-half pound
- Garlic powder, one teaspoon
- Turnip, one medium
- Red beet, one medium
- Thyme, dried, one-half teaspoon
- Extra virgin olive oil, two tablespoons
- Parsnip, one large

Instructions:

Heat the oven to 400. First, you will make the dip by blending all of the listed ingredients together, then cover the dip and refrigerate it until the dip is needed. Mix the garlic powder, thyme, salt, turmeric, and olive oil in a large size mixing bowl. Wash and dry the veggies, and then peel the veggies and slice all of them very thinly. Coat all of the sides of all of the veggies with the oil mix using a pastry brush, and then lay them on a wire rack that you set on top of a baking sheet. Bake the veggie chips for twenty minutes, or a bit longer if you feel it is needed until they are lightly browned and crispy. Serve the chips warm or cool with the dip.

Herbed Cheese Bread

Prep ten min/bake twenty min/serves eight/calories 245

Ingredients:

- Cumin, ground, one-half teaspoon
- Cheddar cheese, shredded, three-fourths cup
- Extra virgin olive oil, one-half cup
- Oregano, dried, one-fourth teaspoon
- Bird's eye chili, minced, one tablespoon
- Thyme, dried, one-fourth teaspoon
- Green onions, finely chopped, one-fourth cup
- Turmeric, ground, one teaspoon
- Garlic, minced, two tablespoons
- French bread, unsliced, one loaf

Instructions:

Heat the oven to 400. Cut the loaf of bread in half from one end to the other end. Fry the green onions, bird's eye chili, and minced garlic for five minutes in the hot oil and then pour the contents of the skillet into a medium-size mixing bowl. Mix in the turmeric, thyme, oregano, and the cumin. Use a knife to spread this mix over the inside halves of the bread. Wrap each of the bread halves loosely in aluminum foil and bake them, with the inside of the bread facing up, for twenty minutes.

Onion Parmesan Arugula Palmiers

Prep ten min/bake fifteen min/makes ten/calories per palmier 189

Ingredients:

- Egg, one beaten
- Red onion, finely chopped, one-half cup
- Puff pastry, one sheet ready-rolled
- Black pepper, one-half teaspoon
- Arugula, chopped, one cup
- Rosemary, dried, one tablespoon
- Parmesan cheese, grated, one fourth cup
- Turmeric, ground, one teaspoon
- Olive oil spray oil

Instructions:

Heat the oven to 400. Lay out the sheet of the puff pastry on a counter or board that has been floured lightly and then cover the sheet of puff pastry with the turmeric, rosemary, arugula, parmesan, pepper, and red onions. Roll the long sides of the pastry up and make them meet in the middle. Use a pastry brush to coat the two sides with the beaten egg and then push the two sides of the pastry sheet together so that they will stick to each other. Use an olive oil spray to coat one baking sheet. Carefully slice the roll into slices that are one-inch thick and then lay the slices on the baking sheet. Bake the palmiers for fifteen minutes.

Tuna Stuffed Avocados

Prep fifteen min/serves two/calories per half of 231

Ingredients:

- Parsley, fresh sliced for garnish
- Avocado, one large unpeeled
- Pesto, two tablespoons
- Tomatoes, minced, two tablespoons
- Black pepper, one-half teaspoon
- Albacore tuna, one can drained
- Black olives, minced, two tablespoons
- Red onions, minced, two tablespoons

Instructions:

Cut the rinsed avocado in down the sides and take out the seed and throw it away. Use a spoon to scrape out half of the flesh from each half. Put the scraped out flesh in a larger mixing bowl. Put in the pesto and the tuna and mash these together well and mix everything all together. Next, add in the red onions, olives, black pepper, and tomatoes and mix well. Spoon the mixture into the avocado shell and sprinkle on the parsley and enjoy.

Loaded Hummus

Prep twenty min/cook twenty-five min/calories thirty per one tablespoon

Ingredients:

- TOPPINGS
- Parsley, fresh chop, two tablespoons
- Cherry tomatoes, one-fourth cup
- Chickpeas, one-fourth cup, crispy
- Walnuts, chopped, two tablespoons
- Red onion, chopped, one-fourth cup
- Celery, minced, one-fourth cup
- Cucumber, chopped, one-fourth cup

- HUMMUS
- Sea salt, one-half teaspoon
- Tahini, two tablespoons
- Chickpeas, one fifteen ounce can drain and rinse
- Black pepper, one teaspoon
- Garlic, minced, one tablespoon
- Extra virgin olive oil, three tablespoons
- Water, four tablespoons
- Paprika, ground, one-half teaspoon
- Lemon juice, one teaspoon
- Turmeric, ground, one-half teaspoon

Instructions:

Heat the oven to 400. Put one-fourth cup of the chickpeas in a shallow oven pan and bake them for twenty-five minutes to make them crispy. Blend all of the rest of the listed ingredients for the hummus until they are smooth and creamy in a blender. Put the hummus onto a platter for serving and arrange the cucumber, celery, onion, and tomatoes on top of the hummus. Garnish with the walnuts, parsley, and crispy chickpeas. Arrange crackers or chunks of pita for dipping.

Fried Goat Cheese With Charred Veggies

Prep ten min/cook fifteen min/serves two/calories 350

Ingredients:

- Goat cheese, four ounces, cut into one-inch pieces
- Extra virgin olive oil, one tablespoon
- Red chicory root, chopped into one-inch pieces, one cup
- Garlic, minced, one teaspoon
- Red onion, one, chopped into large pieces
- Sesame seeds, two tablespoons
- Arugula, four cups, chopped
- Portobello mushrooms, baby, one-half cup sliced
- Walnuts, chopped, two tablespoons
- Red bell pepper, one medium size, cleaned and sliced into eight slices
- Poppy seeds, two tablespoons

Instructions:

Mix together in a medium-size mixing bowl the chopped walnuts, garlic, sesame seeds, and poppy seeds. Place each chunk of goat cheese into this mix to cover both sides completely with the mixture of seeds. Cook the chicory root, pepper slices, onion chunks, and the mushrooms in the hot oil over high heat in a large skillet, charring them on both sides. Put the arugula evenly divided into two serving bowls. Place the charred vegetables in the bowls with the arugula. Add the strips of goat cheese to the skillet and cook them on each side for no more than one minute. Turn these over gently as this cheese will melt quickly. Put the slices of warm cheese in the bowls with the salad and drizzle everything with the olive oil.

**White Bean Kale Dip**

Prep ten min/serves two/calories 269

Ingredients:

- White beans, one fifteen ounce can, drained and rinsed
- Garlic, minced, four tablespoons
- Capers, two tablespoons
- Kale, chopped, two cups
- Extra virgin olive oil, two tablespoons
- Parsley, ground, two tablespoons
- Cayenne pepper, one-half teaspoon
- Lemon juice, two tablespoons

Instructions:

Puree together in a blender the garlic, capers, and white beans (a food processor will also work well for this). Then stir in the kale, cayenne pepper, lemon juice, parsley, and olive oil. Serve this dip with vegetable sticks or toasted pita bread chips.

Roasted Chickpeas

Prep ten min/bake thirty min/serves one/calories 234

Ingredients:

- Chickpeas, two fifteen ounce cans, drain and rinse
- Black pepper, one-half teaspoon
- Turmeric, ground, one teaspoon
- Lemon juice, two teaspoons
- Extra virgin olive oil, two tablespoons
- Parsley, dried, one teaspoon
- Garlic powder, one half teaspoon
- Olive oil spray oil
- Red wine vinegar, two teaspoons

Instructions:

Heat the oven to 425. Pour the chickpeas onto a cookie sheet that you have coated with olive oil spray. Bake the chickpeas for ten minutes, and then stir them and bake them for ten more minutes. Blend the olive oil, turmeric, black pepper, garlic powder, red wine vinegar, parsley, and the lemon juice very well in a medium-sized mixing bowl. After the chickpeas have baked the second time, put them into the bowl of this mix and toss them to coat all of the chickpeas very well. Bake the chickpeas another ten minutes, then let them cool and eat.

Stuffed Artichokes

Prep forty five min/cook thirty min/serves six/calories 325

Ingredients:

- Artichokes, three
- Cottage cheese, low-fat, one half cup
- Red onion, minced, two tablespoons
- Lemon juice, two tablespoons
- Celery, two stalks minced
- Mushroom, chopped, one-half cup
- Sea salt, one teaspoon
- Rosemary, ground, one teaspoon
- Egg, one slightly beaten
- Parsley, chopped, one tablespoon
- Chili sauce, one tablespoon

Instructions:

Heat the oven to 375. Throw away the outside leaves of the artichokes. Cut the inside of the artichokes in half across the middle. Drop the artichoke halves into boiling water and cook them for twenty minutes. Mix together in a medium-size bowl the mushrooms, onions, cottage cheese, egg, lemon juice, chili sauce, parsley, and seasonings and spoon this mixture into the boiled artichoke hearts. Place the filled hearts into a baking pan and bake them for thirty minutes.

Lima Bean Casserole

Prep fifteen min/cook thirty min/serves five/calories 194

Ingredients:

- Lima beans, canned, two cups
- Cheese, mild cheddar, shredded, low fat, one-half cup
- Turmeric, ground, one teaspoon
- Black pepper, one teaspoon
- Lemon juice, two teaspoons
- Extra virgin olive oil, one tablespoon
- Dry mustard, two teaspoons
- Rosemary, dried, one teaspoon
- Tarragon, ground, one teaspoon
- Sea salt, one teaspoon

Instructions:

Heat the oven to 375. Drain the beans and save the liquid. Put the drained beans into an eight by an eight-inch baking pan. Pour in the bean liquid with the olive oil to a skillet and heat well. Add in the turmeric, salt, rosemary, tarragon, pepper, dry mustard, and lemon juice and stir all this together well. Spoon this mixture over the beans in the baking pan and then cover with the shredded cheese. Bake the casserole for thirty minutes.

Okra and Corn Casserole

Prep twenty min/cook thirty min/serves six/calories 135

Ingredients:

- Okra, one pound
- Corn, whole kernel, one can
- Extra virgin olive oil, three tablespoons
- Tomatoes, two large diced
- Sea salt, one half teaspoon
- Black pepper, one teaspoon
- Turmeric, ground, one teaspoon
- Red onion, one small, sliced
- Green bell pepper, one cleaned and sliced
- Garlic, minced, one tablespoon
- Parsley, chopped, one tablespoon

Instructions:

Heat the oven to 375. Cut the okra into bite-sized pieces. Cook the garlic, okra, onion, turmeric, and green pepper in the olive oil for ten minutes. Blend in the parsley and the tomatoes and fry them for ten more minutes. Blend in the corn and pour the entire mixture into a nine by nine-inch baking pan and bake, not covered, for thirty minutes.

Greek Fattoush Salad

Prep fifteen min/serves six/calories 269

Ingredients:

- DRESSING
- Sea salt, one-half teaspoon
- Extra virgin olive oil, one-third cup
- Garlic, minced, two tablespoons
- Red wine vinegar, two tablespoons
- Black pepper, one teaspoon
- Oregano, one-fourth teaspoon

- SALAD
- Sea salt, one-fourth teaspoon
- Red chicory leaves, four cups chop
- Extra virgin olive oil, two tablespoons
- Feta cheese, crumbled, three-fourth cup
- Black olives, one-half cup slice
- Celery, three stalks diced
- Yellow bell pepper, diced
- Parsley, fresh, one-half cup chop
- Arugula, chopped, two cups
- Capers, two tablespoons
- Cherry tomatoes, one cup sliced
- Red onion, one small thinly sliced
- Cucumber, one peeled, quartered and sliced

Instructions:
Put all of the ingredients that are listed for the dressing in a bowl and keep it chilled in the refrigerator until it is time to serve the salad. In a larger size mixing bowl mix the red chicory leaves and the arugula with the celery, bell pepper, olives, tomatoes, capers, cucumber, onion, and parsley, tossing all of the ingredients together gently until they are well mixed. Drizzle on the top the chunks of feta cheese and serve with the dressing on the side.

Chapter 12

The Sirtfood Diet in Real Life

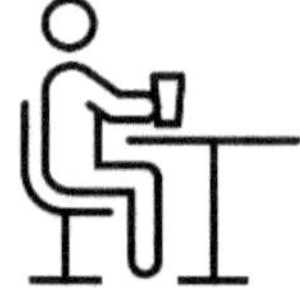

The Sirtfood Diet is easily adapted to any diet plan or life style because you will be eating the foods that you are already accustomed to eating, with sirtfoods added in. This will ensure that you are always consuming a good supply of the sirtuin protein activators that your body will need to keep your sirtuin proteins activated and functioning at their highest level.

Eating Out on the Sirtfood Diet

The Sirtfood Diet is probably the easiest one to take with you because you don't need to rely on any special foods, just load up on plant foods. Any restaurant that serves salads or has a salad bar already has the ingredients you need to make a healthy leafy green salad that is loaded with sirtfoods. If the choice is yours to make, try to pick a vegan-themed restaurant or a buffet style place where you can load your plate with items from the salad section.

As long as most of your meals are eaten at home, you will not need to worry about making any special concessions and you will be able to enjoy an occasional meal out with friends. Add sirtfoods into your regular meals when you eat at home and you will be able to stick to the diet easily.

Eating for Different Nutritional Needs

The needs for certain nutrients for men and women are slightly different. Men should focus more on consuming foods that are loaded with magnesium, fiber, and the vitamins E, C, and B-9. Women should look for those foods that are rich in vitamins D, B-12, and B-6 as well as iron and calcium. The good news about the Sirtfood Diet is that the recommended foods will cover the nutritional needs of both men and women, so there is no need to look for dietary supplements or a different dietary plan. Everyone in the family can consume the same foods, making mealtime more enjoyable.

Eating for Different Body Types

The foods of the Sirtfood Diet will feed every nutritional need that the body has. This means that the foods will provide the best kinds of nutrition whether someone is looking for a long, lean body or they are trying to add on muscles. The foods of the Sirtfood Diet will provide all of the nutrients that anybody will require.

The Sirtfood Diet really is the only eating plan that you will need to follow.

Conclusion

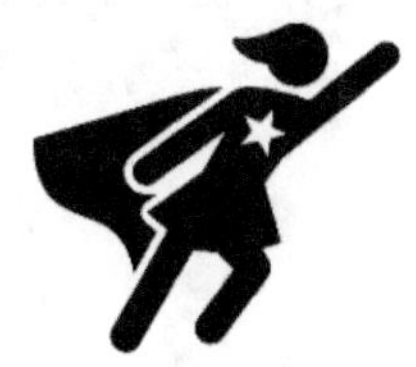

Thank you for making it through to the end of *Sirtfood*. The hope is that it was informative, and you have found all of the tools that you need to help you achieve your goals, whatever they may be.

The next step is to begin your own personal journey into the Sirtfood Diet and start achieving the amazing results that are possible with this diet. Celebrities and athletes all over the world are losing weight and performing great while they are on the Sirtfood Diet. Don't wait any longer to join them and start seeing your own amazing results.

The diet is not difficult to follow, and it is not restrictive. As long as you build your meals around the top sirtuin-containing foods, you will be able to still eat most of the foods that you are consuming now. You will just be adding particular food items to your daily diet, food items that will kick start your skinny gene, and give you the health and appearance you have always wanted.

Finally, if you enjoyed reading this book and found this book helpful in any way, a review on Amazon is always appreciated!